ORGAN DONATION

**Recent Titles in
Health and Medical Issues Today**

ORGAN DONATION

Sarah Boslaugh

Health and Medical Issues Today

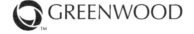

An Imprint of ABC-CLIO, LLC

Santa Barbara, California • Denver, Colorado

This book discusses treatments (including types of medication and mental health therapies), diagnostic tests for various symptoms and mental health disorders, and organizations. The authors have made every effort to present accurate and up-to-date information. However, the information in this book is not intended to recommend or endorse particular treatments or organizations, or substitute for the care or medical advice of a qualified health professional, or used to alter any medical therapy without a medical doctor's advice. Specific situations may require specific therapeutic approaches not included in this book. For those reasons, we recommend that readers follow the advice of qualified health care professionals directly involved in their care. Readers who suspect they may have specific medical problems should consult a physician about any suggestions made in this book.

Library of Congress Cataloging-in-Publication Data

Names: Boslaugh, Sarah, author.
Title: Organ donation / Sarah Boslaugh.
Description: Santa Barbara, California : Greenwood, [2022] | Series: Health and medical issues today | Includes bibliographical references and index.
Identifiers: LCCN 2021032042 (print) | LCCN 2021032043 (ebook) | ISBN 9781440876219 (hardcover) | ISBN 9781440876226 (ebook)
Subjects: LCSH: Donation of organs, tissues, etc. | Transplantation of organs, tissues, etc.
Classification: LCC RD129.5 .B67 2022 (print) | LCC RD129.5 (ebook) | DDC 617.9/54—dc23
LC record available at https://lccn.loc.gov/2021032042
LC ebook record available at https://lccn.loc.gov/2021032043

ISBN: 978-1-4408-7621-9 (print)
        978-1-4408-7622-6 (ebook)

26 25 24 23 22   1 2 3 4 5

This book is also available as an eBook.

Greenwood
An Imprint of ABC-CLIO, LLC

ABC-CLIO, LLC
147 Castilian Drive
Santa Barbara, California 93117
www.abc-clio.com

This book is printed on acid-free paper ∞

Manufactured in the United States of America

Contents

Part III: Scenarios

SERIES FOREWORD

Every day, the public is bombarded with information on developments in medicine and health care. Whether it is on the latest techniques in treatment or research, or on concerns over public health threats, this information directly affects the lives of people more than almost any other issue. Although there are many sources for understanding these topics—from Web sites and blogs to newspapers and magazines—students and ordinary citizens often need one resource that makes sense of the complex health and medical issues affecting their daily lives.

The *Health and Medical Issues Today* series provides just such a one-stop resource for obtaining a solid overview of the most controversial areas of health care in the 21st century. Each volume addresses one topic and provides a balanced summary of what is known. These volumes provide an excellent first step for students and lay people interested in understanding how health care works in our society today.

Each volume is broken into several sections to provide readers and researchers with easy access to the information they need:

Section I provides overview chapters on background information—including chapters on such areas as the historical, scientific, medical, social, and legal issues involved—that a citizen needs to intelligently understand the topic.

Section II provides capsule examinations of the most heated contemporary issues and debates, and analyzes in a balanced manner the viewpoints held by various advocates in the debates.

Section III provides case studies that show examples of the concepts discussed in the previous sections.

A directory of resources and a glossary provide additional reference material and serve as the best next step in learning about the topic at hand.

The *Health and Medical Issues Today* series strives to provide readers with all the information needed to begin making sense of some of the most important debates going on in the world today. The series includes volumes on such topics as stem-cell research, obesity, gene therapy, alternative medicine, organ transplantation, mental health, and more.

PREFACE

Humans have long been fascinated by the possibility of transplanting body parts from one person to another, but not until the second half of the 20th century did organ transplantation became a common part of medical practice. The number of organ transplants performed annually has grown steadily over the decades since, and this lifesaving procedure is now available in many countries of the world. In the United States alone, almost 40,000 organ transplants were performed in 2020, while globally, almost 145,000 transplants were performed in 2018. One major limiting factor in organ transplantation is the availability of suitable donor organs, resulting in over 109,000 people in the United States being wait-listed for a donor organ as of September 2020; sadly, about 17 Americans die each day while waiting for a donor organ.

The process of donation and transplantation is complex and can be confusing, particularly to those who are not professionals in this field. *Organ Donation* offers an overview of the donation and transplantation process, written for nonspecialists, including people needing a transplanted organ, potential donors and their families, and students considering a career related to organ donation and transplantation. While this volume is not intended to replace medical or professional advice, it does offer discussion and clarification of many issues, written for the nonprofessional, that might be of concern to anyone considering becoming involved in the organ donation and transplantation process.

The first section of *Organ Donation* offers an overview of the subject, beginning with an historical summary of how the process of organ transplantation evolved from a theoretical concept to the lifesaving procedure it is today. A statistical summary of organ donation and transplantation today, both in North America and globally, is also provided, as well an overview of pertinent laws. Different types of organ donation are discussed, including deceased and live donation, targeted and untargeted donation, and donation by infants and children as well as adults. The process of organ donation, matching, and transplantation is outlined, with particular emphasis on issues that may be confusing to the nonprofessional, such as how the waiting list for donor organs and the matching process work. The possible experiences of live donors and organ recipients are also discussed, including issues such as organ rejection and the need for immunosuppressive drugs.

Because the process of organ donation and transplantation touches on sensitive topics like body integrity, life, and death, an individual's religious background may affect how they regard organ donation. To help illuminate how organ donation and transplantation are viewed in different religions, *Organ Donation* includes a summary of how these topics are regarded in a variety of religions, including Catholicism, Orthodox Catholicism, different Protestant denominations, Judaism, Islam, Buddhism, and Hinduism. A final chapter in this first section discusses alternatives to organ donation and transplantation, including procedures such as dialysis that can provide support for failing organs, as well as processes intended to increase the supply of available organs, including xenotransplantation, the creation of artificial organs, and organ bioprinting.

The second half of *Organ Donation* covers various controversies in the field, from multiple points of view, with an eye to helping readers clarify their own feelings on these topics. One key topic is the approaches taken in various countries to help meet the unmet need for donor organs. These approaches include switching from an "opt-in" to an "opt-out" system, and organizing campaigns and incentives to encourage people to register as organ donors. Legal issues covered include human organ trafficking, transplant tourism, and the use of organs harvested from prisoners. Financial issues are discussed with a particular eye to the United States, which does not have a national health care system. Ethical issues are also discussed, including different methods of defining death, criticisms of the current organ allocation system, and concerns regarding xenotransplantation and paid organ donation. Finally, five case studies personalize some of the major issues in organ donation and transplantation, while a glossary helps clarify key terms and a bibliography provides the reader with sources that can be used to investigate issues of particular interest in further detail.

PART I

Overview

CHAPTER 1

Organ Donation and Transplantation: Past and Present

Humans have contemplated organ transplantation for thousands of years, at least, but only fairly recently has it become a standard medical procedure offering the recipient a significantly increased life span and improved quality of life. Worldwide, the Global Observatory on Donation and Transplantation (GODT) estimates that over 139,000 solid organ transplants were performed in 2017, with the most common organs transplanted being kidneys (65%) and livers (23%). Despite these impressive numbers, the GODT estimates that currently only about 10% of the need for organ transplants is being met, due to a variety of reasons including an insufficient number of donor organs and the cost and technical demands of organ transplantation.

A HISTORY OF ORGAN DONATION AND TRANSPLANTATION

Discussion of organ transplantation in literary and mythological texts long predates any evidence of actual successful transplantation. For instance, organ transplantation is mentioned in ancient mythology, including sources from Greece, Rome, China, and India. The transplantation of a leg is mentioned in accounts of the Christian martyrs Cosmos and Damien, who lived in what is today Syria in the 3rd century CE. The concept of transplanting a patient's own skin to replace a missing nose is mentioned as early at 600 BCE, and such techniques were used successfully in 16th-century Italy by surgeons such as Gaspare Tagliacozzi. In the 18th century, the Scottish surgeon John Hunter performed experiments in which human teeth were transplanted into a cock's comb, and he suggested that humans could also benefit from tooth transplantation.

The study and practice of organ transplantation in humans became substantially more scientific by the mid-19th century, and reasons for the failures of earlier transplants became better understood. For instance, early attempts at skin grafts were largely unsuccessful because surgeons attempted to transplant full-thickness skin that included layers of fat and other tissues; these extra layers prevented the transplanted skin from developing vascularization. In 1869, the Swiss surgeon Jacques-Louis Reverdin overcame this difficulty by transplanting small "pinch grafts" of a patient's own skin; these small grafts could be used to cover burns and open wounds. The distinction between autografts (using the recipient's own skin) and homografts (using skin from another person) was not generally appreciated during this time, and some surprising claims of successful homographs exist from this period, long before antirejection drugs were available. This may be due to poor record-keeping or complications that interfered with truly observing the results of grafts, because in 1912 Georg Schöne demonstrated convincingly that homografts always failed. Schöne also discovered the "second set" response, which stated that when subsequent homografts from the same donor were performed, each new homograft would fail more rapidly than the previous. Other scientists developed transplant procedures working with animal models, including the French surgeon Alexis Carrel, who performed several successful kidney transplants in dogs. Carrel also developed several important methodologies, including cold graft preservation, and he was awarded the Nobel Prize in Physiology or Medicine in 1912 for this work.

The Ukrainian surgeon U. U. Voronoy, working in the Soviet Union, performed the first human-to-human organ transplant in 1933, a kidney transplant from a deceased donor; however, due to a blood group mismatch between donor and recipient, the patient died two days after the surgery. Voronoy performed several other human transplants over the next two decades, but all failed, and his work did not become well known in the West as it was published only in Russian. Also during the 1930s, Leo Loeb, a German working in the United States, found that lymphocytes were involved in the rejection of homographs, and that genetic disparity between donor and recipient played a role in the rejection of homographs. Sir Peter Medawar, a British biologist who worked with surgeon Thomas Gibson to devise ways to treat burn patients during World War II, made important discoveries in the fields of graft rejection and immune tolerance with skin homografts; he was awarded the Nobel Prize for Physiology or Medicine in 1960 for this work. Gibson and Medawar also reconfirmed that homografts always failed, due to the lack of antirejection medication at the time. The induction of chimerism as an alternative to the use of immunosuppressive drugs was first studied in the 1950s, when Medawar and Billingham discovered that skin could be successfully grafted from one cow to its fraternal twin, due to exchange *in utero* of cells between the twins.

The first successful human-to-human kidney transplant was performed by Joseph Murray in Boston in 1954. Murray got around the problem of graft rejection by transplanting the kidney from one identical twin to another, and the recipient lived for eight years with the transplanted kidney functioning normally. In 1955, Joan Main and Richard Prehn found that using radiation to weaken the immune system of mice, followed by inoculation of bone marrow cells, meant that skin grafts from the bone marrow donor could succeed. Murray used a similar approach with 12 kidney transplant patients in 1958, but all but one of the transplant recipients died. In 1959, Jean Hamburger, working in Paris, was transplanted a kidney from one fraternal (not identical) twin to another following irradiation; the transplant was successful, and the kidney functioned normally until the patient's death from unrelated causes 26 years later.

Dr. Tom Starzl, presenting at a conference in 1963, reported substantially increased success in kidney transplantation using a combination of the drugs azathioprine and prednisone. Other drugs were also tried to suppress the recipient's immune system, including 6-mercaptopurine and steroids, but the true breakthrough came with the discovery of cyclosporine in 1976 and its introduction into clinical use in 1984. Other drugs have since been discovered that are even more effective in suppressing the immune system, and produce fewer side effects, including tacrolinmus, sirolimis, everolimus, and mycophenolic acid.

The introduction of successful methods of immunosuppression spurred the creation of many new renal transplant centers, including 50 in the United States within a year following Starzl's presentation. Dialysis (a method of treating patients with kidney failure) was also developed in this period, and the national medical insurance program Medicare, which previously had served primarily persons over 65, began covering the costs of treatment for patients with end-stage renal disease, regardless of their age. Other innovations in the field of organ transplantation between 1964 and 1980 include the development of antibody screening and tissue typing, the acceptance of brain death as a standard, the development of improved methods to preserve organs after the donor's death, and increased understanding of how to balance the use of immunosuppressive drugs to allow an organ transplant to succeed without also endangering the patient's life due to infection.

The development of improved methods of organ preservation meant that organs could be transported and shared among transplant centers. This fostered the development of networks such as the United Network for Organ Sharing, which managed transplant activities in the United States. At the same time, the lack of sufficient donor organs, relative to the need for them, means that many people each year die waiting for a transplant. A variety of methods have been tried to address this problem, from campaigns to increase voluntary donation to laws in some countries that presume an individual wishes to be an organ donor unless they have indicated otherwise.

ORGAN DONATION AND TRANSPLANTATION TODAY: UNITED STATES

In the United States, according to the Health Resources and Services Administration (HRSA), 36,528 organ transplants were performed in 2018, the highest number ever in one year, and a 5% increase from 2017. Most (81%) of these transplants used organs from a deceased donor, with the remaining 19% using organs from a living donor. Although transplants from a deceased donor remain the most common, the number of living donor transplants has increased over the years, with the 2018 total representing an 11% increase over the number performed in 2017. The number of deceased donors increased 4% from 2017 to 2018, with 10,721 deceased individuals providing at least one organ for transplant in 2018.

Several explanations have been suggested for the increase in donors and transplants, besides improved outreach and medical procedures. One is the increased number of young donors who died from an overdose of opioids, a cause of death that has increased rapidly in recent years. Another possible reason is the broader consideration of who could donate organs, as compared to practices observed in the past. For instance, almost 20% of organs from deceased donors in 2018 came from donors declared dead through circulatory rather than brain death. Another change was the increased use of organs from deceased individuals whose medical profile or other characteristics might make them a less desirable donor. Such individuals include those age 50 or older, those who are considered at heightened risk for a blood-borne disease, and those with an elevated Kidney Donor Profile Index (KDPI) score, the latter indicating that their kidneys may function for less time in the recipient's body than a kidney from a donor with a lower KDPI score. These changes in eligibility represent an effort to balance the desire for each transplant to achieve long-term success with the fact that there remains substantial unmet need for donor organs.

Kidney transplants were the most common type of organ transplant, with 21,167 performed. Second most common were liver transplants, with 8,250, followed by heart transplants (3,408), kidney and pancreas transplants (835), pancreas only transplants (192), intestine transplants (104), and heart and lung transplants (32). Most transplant recipients were Caucasian (55.2%), with smaller numbers being African American (20.6%), Hispanic (16.4%), Asian (5.7%), or other (2.1%); the "other" category includes American Indian/Alaska Native, Pacific Islander, and multiracial. About two-thirds (62%) of organ recipients were male in 2018, with the remaining 38% female.

A total of 17,533 people in the United States donated organs in 2018; of these, 10,722 (61%) were deceased and 6,831 (39%) living. Over one-third (35%) of deceased donors were over the age of 50 and 61% were male. Over two-thirds (65.4%) of the deceased donors were Caucasian, with 16.1% African American, 14.1% Hispanic, 2.3% Asian, and 2.0% other. While persons can donate their organs at any age, the vast majority of donors are working-age adults. In the United States in 2018, according to HRSA, 29.4% of donors were age 18–34 years, 27.5% age 35–49 years, and 27.5% age 50–64 years. In contrast, 1.0% of donors were under the age of one year, 2.1% age 1–5 years, 1.0% age 6–10 years, 4.1% age 11–17 years, and 7.4% over the age of 65.

Over 155 million American are registered as organ donors, representing 58% of American adults. The most common route to register as an organ donor is through a state Department of Motor Vehicles (DMV), where it is typically possible to register as an organ donor while renewing one's driver's license. Montana had the highest rate of registration for organ donation, at 93% of the population, followed by Alaska (92%) and Washington state (89%). The states with the lowest rates of registration for organ donation are New York (32%), Mississippi (37%), and New Jersey (40%). About half (49%) of organs recovered for transplant came from registered donors, along with slightly higher rates of recovered tissues (55%) and recovered eyes (56%); the remaining donations were authorized through consent by family members or next of kin. A high rate of registration is desirable because many people's organs cannot be used for transplantation after their death, so a large number of people need to have indicated their consent for donation in case their organs can be used. The U.S. HRSA estimates that only 3 in 1000 people die in a way that allows their organs to be used for transplantation. HRSA also notes that the most donors in 2018 died of natural causes (43.9%), followed by accidents not caused by motor vehicles (15.6%) and motor vehicle accidents (13.2%).

Despite the increasing number of organ transplants performed in 2018, a substantial waiting list remains for individuals in need of a transplant. As of July 2019, over 113,000 individuals were listed on national transplant waiting lists, including almost 2000 children under age 18; however, most of those on the waiting list are over the age of 50. Just over two-fifths (40.8%) of those on the transplant waiting list are Caucasian, with 28.7% African American, 20.3% Hispanic, 8.2% Asian, and 2.4% other. The most common organ people are waiting for is a kidney (83.7%), followed by a liver (11.6%), heart (3.3%), lung (1.2%), and other organ (1.5%); the "other" category includes pancreas, intestine, and combinations of organs. Note that these figures add to more than 100% because some people are included in multiple categories. Of those who were on the national waiting list in 2018, 62% remained on the waiting list throughout the year, 21% were removed due to receiving a transplant, 3% were removed due to death, and 13% were removed for other reasons.

ORGAN DONATION AND TRANSPLANTATION TODAY: CANADA

According to data from the Canadian Institute for Health Information (CIHI), 2,782 organ transplants were performed in Canada in 2018, representing an increase of 33% since 2009. Organs were transplanted from 762 deceased donors (71% following brain death and 29% following cardiocirculatory death) and 555 from living donors. The deceased donor rate was 20.6 donors per million population, while the living donor rate was 15.0 donors per million population. The most common organ transplanted was a kidney, with 1,706 transplants performed; this was followed by liver transplant (533), lung transplant (361), heart transplant (189), and pancreas transplant (57). Among deceased donors, 60% were male, and an average of 3 organs were used for transplantation from each donor; from deceased donors age 39 and younger, an average of 4 organs per donor were transplanted. Among living donors, 43% were female, and 54% were unrelated to the transplant recipient. The most common organ donated from a living donor was a kidney, which represented 87% of all living donors; the remaining 13% donated part of their liver.

In 2018, 5,900 Canadians (excluding Quebec, due to differences in how records are kept) were living with a liver transplant, and the five-year survival rate for liver transplant patients was 80.9%. In the same year, 2,219 Canadians (excluding Quebec) were living with a transplanted heart, and the five-year survival rate for a heart transplant patient was 85.0%. In addition, Canadians (excluding Quebec) were living with a lung transplant, and the five-year survival rate for lung transplant patients was 66.6%. In 2018, 223 Canadians died while waiting for a transplant, and the waiting list for an organ transplant at the end of 2018 included 4,351 people. Most patients on an organ donation waiting list were waiting for a kidney (3,150), followed by those waiting for a liver (527), lung (270), heart (157), and pancreas (156). Among those who died while waiting for a transplant, most were waiting for a kidney (95) or liver (82), while others were waiting for a lung (28), heart (9), or pancreas (2).

ORGAN DONATION AND TRANSPLANTATION TODAY: AROUND THE WORLD

According to GODT, 139,024 organ transplants were reported in 82 member states of the World Health Organization in 2017. The preponderance of countries included in this report are from Europe, North and South America, and the Middle East; India, Australia, and New Zealand are also included. While this report does not cover every country in the world, it does include most of those in which the preponderance of organ transplants is performed today. In these 82 countries, the most common type of transplant was that of a kidney, with 90,306 kidney transplants being reported; of these, 36.5% were from living donors. The second most commonly transplanted organ was the liver, with 32,348 liver transplants being reported, including 19% from living donors. Other types of transplants reported included heart (7,881), lung (6,084), pancreas (2,243), and small bowel (162).

All 28 member nations of the European Union, representing a population of almost 510 million people, were included in the Global Observatory data. In these countries, a total of 34,221 organ transplants were reported, with the most common type of transplant being that of a kidney: 21,227 kidney transplants were recorded, and 19.9% of these transplants involved a living donor. Second most common was liver transplantation, with 7,940 liver transplants recorded, and 2.8% of those using an organ from a living donor. Other types of transplants reported include heart (2,287), lung (1,980), pancreas (745), and small bowel (42).

The rate of transplantation varied widely from one European Union (EU) country to the next. However, country level should be interpreted while bearing in mind that countries vary widely in population size and that in small countries any statistic with the population as a denominator can change by a large amount from one year to the next due to a relatively small change in the numerator; this effect is even stronger when what is being tracked is a relatively rare procedure such as an organ transplant. However, even among relatively large countries, differences in rates of organ transplantation can be observed. In 2018, the highest rate of patients transplanted was reported in Spain, with a rate of 112.0 per million population; other countries with a relatively high rate of patients transplanted include Belgium (88.8 per million population), Austria (87.7 per million), the Czech Republic (83.4 per million), Croatia (83.6 per million), France (85.8 per million), the United Kingdom (76.9 per million), Portugal (76.0 per million), Romania (76.0 per million), and Sweden (75.3 per million). Countries with the lowest rates of patients transplanted include Bulgaria (6.0 per million), Greece (15.5 per million), and Cyprus (15.8 per million). Several neighboring non-EU countries also had a low rate of transplantation, including Moldova (5.9 per million) and Macedonia (8.1 per million). Thus, it can be seen that the rate of organ transplantation can vary widely among countries in the same part of the world, due to a variety of factors including culture, economics, and national health care priorities.

Not surprisingly, the rate of actual deceased organ donors (donors whose organ(s) were used in transplant) shows a similar pattern to that of the rate of transplantation. Spain had by far the highest rate of actual deceased organ donors in 2018, with 48.3 per million, followed by Portugal (33.4 per million), Belgium (29.9 per million), France (28.8 per million), the Czech Republic (26.6 per million), Estonia (25.4 per million), Austria (24.5 per million), and the United Kingdom (24.3 per million). Cyprus had the lowest rate of actual deceased donors, at 1.7 per million; other countries with comparatively low rates include Bulgaria (2.3 per million), Romania (3.3 per million), and Greece (4.1 per million). Neighboring non-EU countries with relatively low rates of actual deceased organ donors include Macedonia (0.5 per million), Moldova (2.4 per million), and Russia (4.5 per million).

Rates of transplantation for individual organs tend to follow the patterns by country of overall transplantation. For instance, for kidney transplantation, Spain had the highest rate at 71.4 per million population, followed by France (54.7 per million) and the United Kingdom (54.7 per million), and Portugal (48.7 per million). Countries with the lowest rates of kidney transplantation included Bulgaria (3.6 per million population) among European Union (EU countries) and Moldova (3.2 per million) among non-EU European countries.

Australia and New Zealand have moderate to high rates of organ transplantation compared to Europe; however, their relatively small populations (24.8 million for Australia in 2018, 4.7 million for New Zealand) mean that any statistics based on rates should be interpreted with care. In

Australia, 1,780 patients received an organ transplant in 2018, for a rate of 71.8 per million population. Kidney transplants were the most common, with a total of 1,135 performed, for a rate of 45.8 per million population. In New Zealand, a total of 276 patients received an organ transplant in 2018, for a rate of 58.7 per million population. Kidney transplants were the most common, with 182 kidney transplants performed, for a rate of 38.7 per million population.

The rate of overall organ transplantation varied widely across the Latin American countries, according to data from the GODT. Mexico and Uruguay had the highest rate of patients transplanted, at 58.6 per million population, followed by Argentina (47.0 per million population) and Brazil (41.0 per million). Countries with the lowest rates of patients transplanted include Columbia (1.2 per million population), Nicaragua (2.5 per million), and the Dominican Republic (5.2 per million). A similar pattern is seen in the most common type of transplant, that of the kidney. Among the Latin American countries contributing data, rates of kidney transplant are highest in Uruguay (46.0 per million population), Argentina (33.0 per million), Brazil (28.3 per million), and Mexico (23.6 per million) and lowest in Columbia (1.2 per million), Nicaragua (2.5 per million), Peru (4.8 per million), and the Dominican Republic (5.0 per million).

A large number of patients in India received organ transplants in 2018, but relative to the country's large population (1.35 billion), the rate of transplantation is quite low. In 2018, 10,282 patients in India received transplanted organs, for a rate of 7.6 per million population. Kidney transplants were the most common, with 7,936 performed, for a rate of 5.9 per million population. In Saudi Arabia, a total of 1,341 patients received organ transplants, for a rate of 39.9 per million population. Kidney transplants were the most common, with 1,006 performed in 2018 for a rate of 29.9 per million. In Kuwait, 74 patients received organ transplants in 2018, for a rate of 17.6 per million population. Kidney transplants were the most common, with 70 being performed, for a rate of 16.7 per million population.

LAWS REGULATING ORGAN DONATION AND TRANSPLANTATION: UNITED STATES

In the United States, the process of organ donation and transplantation is highly regulated, with multiple agencies involved and relevant regulations existing at both the federal (national) and state level. Primary oversight in the field of organ donation and transplantation is granted to a federal agency, HRSA, which exists within the U.S. Department of Health and Human Services. Other federal agencies that play key roles in the organ donation and transplantation process include the Centers for Medicare and Medicaid Services (CMS), the Centers for Disease Control and Prevention (CDC), the National Institutes of Health (NIH), the Agency for Healthcare Research and Quality (AHRQ), and the Food and Drug Administration (FDA).

The primary legislation governing organ donation in the United States is the *Uniform Anatomical Gift Act* (UAGA), a piece of model legislation written by law and policy experts in 1968, which has been revised and updated since then. The UAGA was offered to each state for adoption, with the aim of producing consistency in the organ donation process across the nation. Due to the reserved powers of each state as specified in the U.S. Constitution, many matters regarding organ donation, including those regarding contracts, gifting, and public health, cannot be directly specified at the federal level, but must be established through state law. The use of model legislation is a method to create consistency at the national level in matters related to organ donation, while still giving each state power over its own laws and regulations. The UAGA, which in its original form has in fact been adopted by every state, is an "opt-in" law, meaning that an individual or his or her next of kin must make a voluntary and affirmative declaration of the intent to donate organs at the time of death.

Organ donation in the United States, under the UAGA, is governed by the principles of gift law. Legally speaking, a gift is the voluntary and legally binding transfer, without payment, of something from one person to another. Ordinary contract law does not apply to organ donation because the United States prohibits the sale or purchase of organs, and contract law requires a "consideration" (something of value, i.e., a payment) be made in exchange for the promise of the transfer of something from one party to another. A donated organ is considered to be transferred from the donor to the recipient, which allows others involved in the organ donation process (e.g., doctors and nurses) to be paid for their work in facilitating the transfer. The doctrine of informed consent, which governs most medical procedures and research, does not apply to organ donation from deceased donors for two reasons: first, because the procedure provides neither risks nor benefits to the individual donating (as they are already dead at the time of donation), and second, because permission for donation is often provided many years in advance of the person's death, making it impossible to know the details of the donation in advance (e.g., which organs, if any, will actually be donated). For this reason, the language of "authorization" rather than "consent" is used in a legal context with organ donation: an individual authorizes an anatomical gift when they sign up to be an organ donor.

A legally binding transfer of a gift requires three elements: (1) donative intent, meaning that the donor intends to make the gift, (2) transfer from the donor to the recipient, and (3) acceptance by the recipient. The UAGA provides two ways to authorize donation: the individual may do so prior to his or her death, or a surrogate (e.g., the individual's next of kin or other family member) may do so after the individual's death. In the first method, known as first-person authorization, typically a person registers their intent through a donor registry. If an individual indicates their consent to donate upon their death, this is legally binding and cannot be revoked by family members. In the second method, if an individual's organs are medically eligible for donation (which is true in only a small fraction of deaths) and the individual has not previously indicated their consent to donate, the surrogate may be approached and asked to give permission for the deceased's organs to be donated.

The original version of the UAGA was written in 1968 to increase organ donation in the United States; publicity followed the first successful heart transplant the previous year. This widely publicized successful transplant increased public awareness of the lifesaving potential of organ transplantation and the need for more donors and may have helped motivate creation of this law. The UAGA established gift law as the legal principle governing organ donation in the United States and established an individual's explicit desire to donate their organs upon death as sufficient for the exchange to take place. The first version of the UAGA was adopted by all U.S. states, in the process replacing many conflicting and inconsistent state laws; however, subsequent revisions of the UAGA were not adopted by all states.

In 1987, the UAGA was revised to explicitly prioritize the donor's wishes over that of the next of kin or other family members so that an individual's wish to donate their organs after death could not normally be overruled by objections from family members. Other stipulations included in the 1987 revision were the definition of a bodily organ or other body part as property, establishment of a uniform set of procedures for obtaining an individual's authorization for organ donation, and the stipulation that organ donation could not be used to obstruct an autopsy or coroner's investigation. A second revision in 2006 allowed individuals to register their desire to donate by many different means, including expressing this wish when obtaining a driver's license, including it in a will or advance directive, registering with a state donor registry, or expressing it verbally. Language strengthening the right of an adult to choose whether to donate or not was also added (although parents could still overrule the wishes of a minor child). The 2006 revision also made it a felony to buy or sell human body parts or to destroy or falsify organ donor documentation and prioritized the use of organs for transplantation or therapy over their use for research.

In the case of organ donation from a living donor, additional considerations are relevant because the health and recovery of the donor is a matter of concern. Because health insurance is provided by a variety of different sources in the United States, and in many cases is regulated at the state rather than federal level, it is difficult to generalize about the laws governing living donation (independent of those laws governing all organ donation). The federal government provides 30 days of paid leave for living organ donors and 5 days for bone marrow transplantation, above and beyond an individual's annual sick leave and vacation time. Some states also require that employees be granted leave of a certain length for serving as a living organ donor; these benefits may apply only to state employees, or to both state and private sector employees, and the leave may be paid or unpaid. The federal government provides no tax breaks for living organ donors, not even a charitable deduction, because that would require placing a dollar amount on the value of the donation. However, some states provide an organ donation tax deduction, ranging from a few hundred dollars to ten thousand dollars, to cover unreimbursed expenses related to organ donation, including travel, lodging, medical expenses, and lost income; the details of what is covered, and the amount allowed, vary from one state or another.

Laws Regulating Organ Donation and Transplantation: Other Countries

Laws regarding organ donation vary widely from one country to another and may also differ within different parts of the same country. For instance, in one country it may be illegal to buy or sell a human organ, while in another country organ sale is permitted and is administered by the government. In some countries, organ transplantation is included within the national framework of health insurance or health care, while in others it is not. In some countries, organ donation and transplantation is administered at the national level, while in other countries, these responsibilities are managed at the state or provincial level. In some countries, a supernational organization such as the European Union creates regulations that are nationally binding for each member country, while in other countries such as the United States, the laws determining organ donation and transplantation are determined entirely within the country.

In the EU, the legal framework governing organ transplantation is stated in the *European Organs Directive*, also known as *Directive 2010/53/EU*. This directive entered into force on August 26, 2010, and EU countries were required to incorporate it into their national legislation by August 27, 2012. This directive covers organ donation, testing, procurement, preservation, characterization, transport, and transplantation; seeks to ensure that uniform quality, safety and legal standards will apply to donors and recipients; and includes rules to ensure quality and safety standards for organ transplantation. The *European Organs Directive* requires member nations to create a quality and safety framework for the organ chain from donation to transplantation, requires that donor selection and evaluation be carried out by recognized personnel and organizations, and provides specific detail on matters such as the data that must be made available about donors and regulations regarding organ transport. It also specifies that organ procurement and transplant must take place in authorized centers and that systems must be created to allow tracing from donor to recipient, and recipient to donor, for at least 30 years. The directive also requires that countries create a system to report and investigate adverse reactions, to share information when organs cross country boundaries, to carefully select and screen living donors, to ensure that all donations are voluntary and unpaid, to protect the personal data of donors and recipients, and to exchange information through the network created by the European Commission.

In Canada, national legislation governs the safety of donated organs, while all other aspects of organ donation and transplantation are governed by the laws of each province or territory. In 2001, the Canadian Council for Donation and Transplantation was created to serve as an advisory body to the Conference of Deputy Ministers of Health, to coordinate activities related to the donation and transplantation of organs at the federal, provincial, and territorial level. In 2007, these duties were transferred to Canadian Blood Services, which expanded its scope to include donation of organs and tissues as well as blood. Also in 2007, federal regulations governing the organ donation process came into effect; these regulations covered matters such as the determination of donor suitability and establishing exclusionary criteria for donors. Those exclusionary criteria include HIV infection, death from unknown causes, infection with a prion disease, and behaviors that place the individual at a high risk for HIV and viral hepatitis.

Canada does not have a national donor database or national waiting list for all donated organs; instead, each province or territory maintains its own registries. The Living Donor Paid Exchange, renamed the Kidney

Paired Donation Program in 2014, lists pairs of individuals—one willing to donate a kidney, the other in need of a donated kidney—and aims to match pairs on the basis of blood group and tissue type to facilitate transplants. Over 500 kidney transplants were facilitated through this program between 2009 and 2017. The National Organ Waitlist (NOW), created in 2012, is a secure database of Canadians waiting for transplant of any organ but the kidney; provincial and territorial transplantation programs can access the NOW database to identify potential organ recipients in critical need anywhere in Canada. The Highly Sensitized Patient Program, created in 2013, lists kidney transplant patients who are difficult to match due to a highly sensitized immune system; it has facilitated 368 kidney transplants since 2013. The OneMatch Stem Cell and Marrow Registry lists potential donors of bone marrow and peripheral blood for all provinces except Quebec; in Quebec, the Stem Cell Donor Registry serves the same purpose.

As of 2018, all Canadian provinces and territories required explicit consent for donation after death. However, in 2019 the possibility of adopting presumed consent (an "opt-out" rather than "opt-in" system) was discussed in several provinces, and in April, Nova Scotia became the first province to adopt an "opt-out" system. In November 2019, Alberta became the second province to adapt an "opt-out" system. However, the system adopted was a "soft opt-out" program in which an individual would be presumed to be a donor unless they had specified otherwise, but permission of their family or next of kin would be required before donation could take place. As of 2018, all provinces but Saskatchewan linked a donor's intent to donate with their health cards and/or driver's licenses, and British Columbia, Alberta, Manitoba, and Ontario have web-based donor registries to facilitate an individual indicating their intent to donate their organs after death.

While a black market in human organs exists in multiple countries, Iran is unique (as of 2020) in allowing the legal sale of kidneys. The process is regulated through a government-run agency, the Kidney Foundation of Iran. An individual who wishes to sell their kidney registers with the Foundation, which tries to match them with a compatible recipient. The price for a donated kidney is fixed (the equivalent of US$4,600 in 2017), and the government pays for the surgery, which must be performed at a government hospital. Private sale of a kidney or other organ is banned by law, and the current system was developed in part to bring some control over the process of donation and sale of organs. However, there is evidence that private sales continue, in part because a private buyer may be willing to pay much more than the official price. According to the Iranian government, their system that allows the legal sale of kidneys has nearly eliminated the waiting list for kidney transplants in Iran.

In Israel, the current organ transplant law was passed in 2008 in an attempt to clarify how death would be determined and to respond to several social problems, including a lack of available organs for transplant, and the growth of organ trafficking and transplant tourism. This law establishes brain death as a legal standard of death, a common standard internationally but one that conflicts with the beliefs of the ultra-Orthodox Jewish community. Unlike the laws in many countries, Israeli law grants the most favored access to donated organs to individuals who are donors and to the first-degree relatives of donors, followed by individuals registered as donors, and finally first-degree relatives of persons registered as donors. Consent for donation is opt in, and consent of family members is required even for deceased donors who have clearly indicated their desire to donate their organs upon death.

People have long contemplated the possibility of transferring organs or other body parts from one person to another, but only fairly recently have organ transplants become a standard and lifesaving medical procedure. Although over 139,000 organs were transplanted worldwide in 2017, this number does not begin to meet the need for transplants. Even in rich and technologically advanced countries like the United States, people die every year while waiting for a donated organ, and in poorer countries, receiving an organ transplant is not even a remote possibility for most of the population. Countries differ in the ways they regulate organ donation and transplantation, including matters such as whether organs may be bought and sold, what level of government is in charge of the system of procuring and allocating organs, and what systems are used to determine who has priority in allocating donated organs.

CHAPTER 2

Types of Organ Donation

Although it is common to think of organ donation as a single process, in fact there are many different types of organs and tissues that may be donated. The sources of organs also differ, as do the processes by which donated organs enter the allocation system and are assigned to recipients. When the donor is a minor, or when a donation is received from a newborn child, additional issues arise. Finally, donated organs can be used in medical research as well as for transplantation, although the needs of transplantation are generally given the highest priority. These specificities and details are important in understanding how the organ donation process works.

WHAT TISSUES AND ORGANS CAN BE DONATED

A broad range of human organs and tissues can be donated and successfully transplanted. While the difference between organs and tissues may not be obvious to the layman, in biology, a distinction is made between them. Tissues represent a lower level of organization and are made up of similar types of cells, while organs represent a higher level of organization, are made up of similar types of tissues, and perform specific functions in the body such as breathing or pumping blood. Human organs that can currently be donated by a deceased donor include the kidneys, the liver, the lungs, the heart, the pancreas, and the intestines. Living donors can donate a single kidney; a single lung; or part of their lungs, liver, pancreas, or intestine. It is also possible to donate body tissues (such as the cornea) and complex body parts such as the hands or the face.

An individual can donate their corneas and sclera (both considered body tissue rather than organs) to be used for transplant after death. The cornea is the clear part of the eye that covers the iris and pupil, and a corneal transplant can replace an individual's cornea that has become diseased or scarred, as from eye disease, injury, or birth defects. Unlike most organ transplants, corneas do not need to be matched to the recipient, and matters such as blood type, age, eye color, or quality of eyesight have no bearing on whether a transplant will be successful or not. Also, unlike most organ donations, the cornea can be recovered from a donor several hours after death and can be stored for up to 14 days and still transplanted successfully into a recipient. Most individuals can donate their corneas, the exception being individuals with infections or a few diseases including HIV. The sclera, the white part of the eye surrounding the pupil, can also be donated and can be used in operations to rebuild the eye.

Many body tissues can be transplanted from donor to recipient and can save or improve the quality of life of the donor; in fact, combining tissue and organ donation, a single donor can save or enhance the lives of up to fifty people. Besides corneas and the sclera, skin, bone, tendons, heart valves, and other body tissues can be donated after death. Most people can be tissue donors even if they cannot be organ donors, and although tissue donation must begin within 24 hours of the donor's death, tissues can be stored for use for some time after removal from the donor. Donated heart valves can be used to repair the hearts of both children and adults whose heart valves have been damaged due to birth defects or other causes. Donated skin can be used to cover burned areas on another person's body, thus acting as a lifesaving shield against infection. Donated bone can be used to replace bone removed from the recipient's body due to illness or injury or used as part of the process to implant artificial joints in people. Donated tendons can also be used to rebuild damaged joints in the recipient's body.

Transplantation of entire hands, arms, or faces is a relatively new process within the field of organ donation and transplantation. Surgery to replace an arm, hand, or face is called a vascularized composite allograft or Vascularized Composite Allograft (VCA) organ transplant, because the process requires grafting many types of tissue, including bone, muscle, nerves, skin, and blood vessels. Although hand and face transplants are the most common type of VCA organ transplant, other body parts including the larynx, abdominal wall, and genitalia have also been transplanted. Rejection is an issue in VCA organ transplantation, and the same types of matching must be done with a VCA organ transplant as with any organ transplant. Additional factors must also be matched for some VCA transplants, such as skin color and tone, body size, and gender. VCA transplants remain relatively rare, due to the complexity of the process and the recent development of the necessary techniques—the first hand transplant was performed in 2005, the first face transplant in 2007—and as of January 2018, fewer than 200 VCA transplants have been performed worldwide.

Individuals can also donate blood stem cells, which come from three sources: blood marrow, the umbilical cord, and peripheral blood stem cells. Bone marrow is the soft tissue in the interior cavity of bones; most blood is produced there, and some of the marrow may be removed to obtain stem cells. Living donors can contribute bone marrow through a surgical procedure in which liquid marrow is removed from the pelvic bone using needles. The umbilical cord also contains high levels of blood stem cells, and cord blood can be collected and stored for long periods of time. Peripheral blood stem cells can be created by injecting a donor with the drug filgrastim, which increases the number of stem cells circulating in the blood stream. These stem cells, which are the same type as those collected from the bone marrow, can be collected through a process similar to blood donation. Matching is necessary between a blood stem cell donor and recipient, and donors must be healthy and between the ages of 18 and 60.

DECEASED AND LIVE DONATION

Organs can be successfully transplanted after being donated from either deceased or live donors. Most donated organs today come from deceased donors, and far more organs can be used from a deceased than from a live donor, but the practice of live donation is increasing. The process by which one becomes a deceased donor varies depending on the laws of the country, including whether an "opt-in" or "opt-out" system is in use. In an opt-in system, which is used in the United States, a person must explicitly state their desire to be an organ donor before death, often by stating this desire on a public registry. If a person has not expressed such a desire, his or her next of kin may be approached by hospital staff and asked if they would like to donate their loved one's organs, but there is no presumption that a person wishes to donate if they have not explicitly stated that desire. In an opt-out system, everyone is presumed to be willing to donate their organs after death, unless they have explicitly stated that they do not wish to do so. Some European countries and Canadian provinces have adopted an opt-out system, but generally require the permission of the deceased individual's next of kin or other family members before proceeding with the donation process (a so-called "soft op-out" process).

Far more people are registered as organ donors than will ever actually donate organs for transplantation, primarily because a deceased donor must die in specific circumstances for their organs to be usable. A patient receives the same medical care whether or not they are registered as a donor; that is, everything possible will be done to save their life, including placing them on life support if necessary. Only after brain death (the cessation of all brain activity) has occurred will the fact that a person is a potential donor becomes relevant. If the person's organs are eligible for donation, local, regional, or national networks will begin the process of matching the donor organs to individuals registered as needing a transplant; in the United States, this process is handled by the Organ Procurement and Transplantation Network (OPTN). Organs donated after death typically go to the recipient who is the best match for the organ and who is likely to be unknown to the person donating the organ and their family. The method of allocating donated organs differs in each country, but in the United States, most donated organs are allocated to patients within the same region, while some are allocated to patients in other parts of the country.

Live organ donation is possible for only a few organs, and often a living donation is targeted, meaning that the organ in question is meant for a particular recipient. For instance, someone might choose to donate a kidney to a family member suffering from kidney failure. Living donation is limited to organs that can be removed while allowing the donor to continue living a fully functioning life. These organs include a single kidney (because the donor can live a healthy life with only one functioning kidney), part of the liver (because the liver can regenerate in the donor's body), a lung or part of a lung (because the donor can live with only one lung), and part of the pancreas or intestines (because a person can live a healthy life with only part of their pancreas or intestines). Some tissues can also be donated by living donors, often after they have been removed in the course of medical procedures. For instance, skin removed in the course of an abdominoplasty (tummy tuck) can be donated, as can bone removed during knee or hip replacement. Bone marrow can be donated by a living donor, because it is regenerated in the donor's body, and the amnion and blood from the umbilical cord can be donated after childbirth.

The health and well-being of the donor, and the potential effects of the donation, are a factor in determining whether live donation is possible. In general, a donor must be a match to the recipient and must also be an adult (age 18–60) in good health and not suffering from a chronic condition such as diabetes, high blood pressure, kidney disease, heart disease, or cancer (organ donation by those under age 18 is discussed later). Surgery itself also poses risks, and a small percentage of donors have suffered complications due to donation. Living donation is a relatively recent practice, and the potential long-term costs to the donor are not entirely known.

However, research is currently being conducted to determine if there are any long-term effects on donor health to living donation—for instance, if donating one kidney places greater strain on the remaining kidney. In the United States, individuals considering becoming a donor must also consider how this choice will impact their future ability to obtain health insurance, because we do not have a system of universal health care or health insurance coverage.

Living organ donation allows a patient waiting for an organ to bypass the waiting list for a suitable organ from a deceased donor. In addition, living donor organ transplants are associated with longer survival of the organ and fewer complications than with transplants from deceased donors. The Center for Liver Disease and Transplantation at the Columbia University Irving Medical Center reports that the three-year survival rate for adult liver patients receiving a living donor liver is 96.7%, as compared to 78.9% for patients receiving a liver from a deceased donor. For pediatric patients, the three-year survival rate with a liver transplant from a living donor is 100%, as compared to 97% for a patient with a liver transplant from a deceased donor. Hypothesized reasons from the improved survival and function of living donor organs include the shorter waiting time for an organ and optimal timing for the transplantation. The operation to remove and transplant the liver can be planned in advance, and a liver from a living donor can be transplanted immediately after being removed from the donor.

Living donors may take part in paired organ donation or a donation chain, In paired organ donation, also known as paired exchange, a donor may not be able to donate to an intended recipient due to differences in blood or tissue type, but may be able to donate to someone else who is paired with a donor who can donate to the first recipient. In this way, both donors can give their organ to someone who is compatible to receive it, and both recipients can receive an organ matched to them. A living organ donation chain is similar but on a larger scale: a donor donates an organ to a recipient, who is paired with a donor who donates to a second recipient, who is paired with a donor who donates to a third recipient, and so on, with each donor-recipient pair matched for compatibility.

TARGETED AND UNTARGETED DONATION

When a person chooses to donate one or more organs, they may make either a targeted or untargeted donation. In a targeted donation, the donor specifies that the organ will go to a specific recipient. Targeted donation is common when the organ comes from a living donor, and often the recipient is a relative or close friend of the donor. A living donor may also make an untargeted donation, also known as an altruistic or good Samaritan donation, in which case the donor does not know the recipient. In this type of untargeted donation, the donor and recipient may decide to meet if both agree and it is allowed by the transplant center.

In contrast, most deceased organ donations are untargeted—the donor simply indicates that their organs may be removed after their death, and the system of organ allocation in use in their geographical area determines who receives the organ. Deceased organ donations are usually anonymous, meaning that the donor and the donor's family do not know the recipient or the recipient's family. However, sometimes donor and recipient families may arrange to meet if both agree to this arrangement and if it is allowed by the organ transplant center.

ORGAN DONATION BY MINORS

Most organ donors are adults, who can legally give consent for their organs to be donated. However, children under the age of 18 can also donate their organs if specified conditions are met, and often the recipients of these organs are other children. In the case of donation after death, the parents or other next of kin of the child generally can choose to donate their child's organs or not. While in some states it is possible for a person younger than 18 to sign up as an organ donor when that person receives his or her driving learner's permit or driver's license, permission of the individual's parents is generally required for donation if he or she dies before the age of 18. Some children have also served as living organ donors, but because of the potential risks to the donor, this type of donation is usually approved only in very specific circumstances. In the United States in 2018, over 800 children under the age of 18 were organ donors, and over 1,800 children received organ transplants (from both pediatric and adult donors). Most child organ donors in 2018 were between the ages of 11 and 17, but over 100 were less than 1 year old.

Organs for transplant frequently need to be matched to the size of the recipient, so a child needs a child-sized organ. This is a principal reason organs from children are sought for donation. In some cases, it is also possible to transplant a portion of an adult organ, such as a liver or lung, into a child. Most children under age of one year on the organ waiting list are waiting for a donor liver or a heart. Children ages 1–10 are most commonly waiting for a donor kidney or liver, followed by a heart, while those age 11–17 are most commonly waiting for a kidney, followed by a liver. Some highly publicized cases of children whose organs have been donated, such as that of Nicholas Green, an Anglo-American boy who was killed in Italy, have aided the cause of organ donation by helping people to realize how many lives can be saved by the organs of a single donor, and that children as well as adults can donate organs.

Children have successfully donated kidneys and bone marrow at numerous transplantation centers. Usually such donors are between the ages of 16 and 18, and an extensive medical and psychological workup is performed before the transplant is granted. These precautions are necessary to be certain that the donor is a good match, that they understand the possible consequences of being a living donor, and that they have reached the decision to donate through their own freewill, without being pressured by family members or anyone else. The most common cases in which living organ donation by a minor is approved by a transplant center include when there is a very close match between donor and recipient (for instance, when the donation is from one identical twin to the other), when the risk to the donor's future health and well-being is judged to be extremely low, and when there is no other good opportunity for a suitable organ; in any case, it must be entirely clear that the minor has not been coerced into agreeing to donate.

NEONATAL DONATION

A newborn child is called a neonate, from the Latin terms for "new" and "birth." The term "neonate" is usually used to refer to a child from birth until four weeks of age, although sometimes it is used to refer to children up to two months old. Children who die as neonates can donate organs and tissues that are suitable for transplant or may be used for medical research. The responsibility for donation lies with the parents, of course, and they may be approached by a representative of an organ procurement organization similarly to the way that a representative would approach anyone whose loved one is a potential deceased donor. The field of neonatal organ and tissue donation and transplantation is much younger than that of organ donation and transplantation from adults or older children, and the study of donation during this early period of life is also complicated by the fact that often official statistics concerning donors are not broken down into age groups smaller than one year, so special research is required to get information about neonatal donors. However, studies looking at the potential for organ donation following death in the neonatal period, such as that by Michelle Labrecque and colleagues, have found that a significant number of organs can be recovered from neonates if standard donation procedures are followed.

There are special concerns regarding donation from very young children, beginning with the difficulty of determining brain death in children with immature brain stem reflexes. The law in some countries effectively precludes the possibility of donation by very young children or may complicate efforts to encourage donation at that age. For instance, K. C. Hawkins and colleagues note that prior to 2015, brain stem death was not an accepted diagnosis in small infants in the United Kingdom, although organs from children whose death was determined by that standard in other countries could be imported into the country and used for transplantation. In April 2015, an expert commission produced guides for the diagnosis of death using neurological criteria for children under two months of age, thus creating the possibility for children of this age to donate organs after brain stem death. Prior to this change, only infants whose death was confirmed by circulatory criteria could donate organs; in practice, this standard was applied primarily to infants born with anencephaly (absence of much of the brain and skull due to a neural tube defect; children with this condition typically live only a few hours or days after birth). In 2015 and 2016, only six children under the age of two months were actual organ donors in the United Kingdom: one became a donor after neurological determination of death, the other five after circulatory determination of death.

Matthew J. Weiss and colleagues note that because the death of a young child is by definition a tragedy, physicians may be reluctant to refer parents of child patients to the local organ donation organization, resulting in many lost opportunities to donate. For instance, one study found that clinicians fail to refer parents to the local organ procurement organization in 23% of cases in which life-sustaining therapy has been withdrawn from a child, with an even higher rate of non-referral (39%) for patients age from one week to one month. This lack of referrals is contrary to the principles advocated by most organ donation organizations, which encourage clinicians to refer children to the local organ procurement organization in all cases of neurologic injury that may lead to brain death or when the decision has been made to withdraw life-sustaining therapy. The discussion of donation must be sensitive to the feelings of the parents and conducted separately from delivering the news of the child's prognosis, and parents must be informed about the donation process and given sufficient time to reach a decision.

ORGAN DONATION FOR MEDICAL RESEARCH

Transplantation may be the use that first comes to mind when discussing organ donation, but donated organs can also be used in medical research, where scientists can use them to help develop treatments that will save lives in the future. For instance, islet cell transplantation, a treatment for Type I diabetes in which islet cells taken from the pancreas are reproduced in the liver, was developed with the use of donated organs. This method of treatment can effectively cure Type I diabetes so that people who formerly suffered from that disease no longer need insulin shots. Other examples of diseases where research has been aided by donated organs and tissue include glaucoma, diabetic retinopathy, age-related macular generation, coronary artery disease, viral hepatitis, cirrhosis, cystic fibrosis, and pulmonary hypertension.

While transplantation is the first priority for donated organs and tissues, criteria for organs acceptable for research are lower than those used for transplantation, and often organs from older donors or from individuals with diseases that would otherwise disqualify them from donating for transplantation can be used gainfully in a research setting. In addition, the range of organs and tissues that can be used in research is broader than those that can currently be transplanted, and nearly every organ system in the body includes organs and tissues that can be used for research. The International Institute for the Advancement of Medicine (IIAM) works with organ procurement organizations in the United States to identify donated organs that are not suitable for transplant and to get them to organizations that can use them in research. In 2012, the IIAM established a Neonatal Donor Program. As of December 2019, the IIAM had received 478 neonatal donations from 131 families.

Many different types of organs and tissues may be donated today, and donated organs may be used in medical research as well as for transplantation. Organs may be obtained from a wide variety of donors as well—for instance, while most donors are adults, organs have also been successfully transplanted from children under one year of age. While most organs for transplantation are obtained from deceased donors, living donors provide an increasing percentage of organs, and often participate in targeted donation, in which the organ is specified to go to a particular person. Special considerations apply when a living person chooses to donate an organ, because the potential effect on their health must be considered as well as the expected benefits to the recipient. When the donor is a child, additional considerations also apply, in particular if a living donation is being contemplated. These specificities and details are important in understanding how the organ donation process works and when considering whether the current system should or could be changed.

CHAPTER 3

The Process of Organ Donation, Matching, and Transplantation

Organ donation and transplantation is a complex process. While it is understandable to focus on the end result—lives saved due to successful organ transplantation—it's also worth considering all the steps that need to happen before arriving at that point. The preliminary aspects of a successful organ transplantation include a potential donor indicating their willingness to donate, the person who needs an organ being placed on a waiting list, the needed organ becoming available, a match being made between a donor and a recipient, and the organ in question being transported to the site where the transplantation will take place; only then can the organ be transplanted into the recipient. In most countries, including the United States, the demand for donated organs far exceeds the supply, so decisions have to be made about who gets each available organ, adding another layer of complexity to the process. Because the donation and matching process differs from one country to the next, this chapter will concentrate on how this process is carried out in the United States.

BECOMING AN ORGAN DONOR

In the United States, people who wish to become organ donors typically add their names to a donor registry. Joining such a registry means you have given legal permission for the anatomical donation of your organs, tissues, and eyes. Because most American adults visit their local Bureau of Motor

Vehicles (BMV) office at least once every few years, for purposes such as renewing their driver's license or paying their vehicle registration fees, BMV offices in the United States have forms available for individuals to register as organ donors. People who have signed up for a donor registry in this way can usually have this fact indicated on their driver's license. The paperwork to become an organ donor is also available on the internet, or from any of the 58 Organ Procurement Organizations in the United States. Although it is not legally required, it is also a recommended practice for a donor to let his or her family know that they have indicated their desire to become an organ donor, so that information does not come as a surprise to the family and they do not oppose the donor's will following the donor's death.

Nearly any person is a potential organ and tissue donor, should they elect to be one. When a person dies, a medical evaluation is performed to determine which, if any, organs from the deceased individual are suitable for transplant. A few conditions totally disqualify an individual from organ and tissue donation, so there is no need for a potential donor to preemptively disqualify themselves from donation. In 2019, one out of three people who donated organs in the United States were over the age of 50, and organs have been successfully transplanted from people over the age of 90. Persons under the age of 18 can also be organ donors, although usually the donation must also be authorized by the minor's legal guardian. In some states, persons younger than 18 can register as organ donors at the time they get their learner's permit or driver's license, but if they die before reaching age 18, the legal guardian would still need to give permission for the donation to be carried out. In 2019, over 900 individuals under the age of 18 were organ donors in the United States.

People are sometimes concerned that if they are registered as an organ donor, they will not receive optimal medical care or that a full effort will not be made to save their life. However, this belief is not correct, and a patient's status as an organ donor does not influence the quality of medical care they will receive. To put it another way, everyone working within the medical system will make the same effort to save the life of an individual under their care, whether or not that individual is registered as an organ donor. Organ donation only becomes a consideration after a person has died and cannot be revived. Most often, death in this context is determined by brain death, which means that a person has no brain activity and is unable to breathe on his or her own. A person who has suffered brain death cannot be revived and will be officially recorded as dead; only after this point does organ donation become possible.

GETTING ON THE TRANSPLANT WAITING LIST

Because the need for donated organs far exceeds the supply, individuals needing an organ transplant typically register their name on a waiting list. As with any scarce resource, particularly one that could make the difference between life and death, difficult choices may have to be made concerning who receives an available organ and who doesn't, and sometimes decisions about allocating organs are controversial.

A person may know that they will need an organ transplant before that need becomes critical. For instance, they may have a progressive disease that is predicted to eventually cause organ failure or a birth defect that is predicted to result in organ failure in the future. The process of getting on the organ donation list begins with a referral from the patient's physician, followed by evaluation at an organ transplant center. All transplant centers in the United States are part of the OPTN, and it is possible to research different centers before choosing the one at which a patient will be evaluated. Considerations involved in choosing a center include the center's expertise in the specific type of transplant needed, the location of the center, and financial considerations including how compatible the patient's health insurance is with the demands that will be placed on it during the transplantation process.

Once a transplant center is selected, the individual needing the transplant will register for an evaluation appointment, during which time they will learn if they are a good candidate for transplant. This evaluation will include medical tests and a psychological evaluation to see if the individual meets the center's criteria to be a transplant candidate. The transplant evaluation is also a good opportunity for the transplant candidate to meet with members of the transplant team and become more familiar with the transplant center. The decision to accept or reject a candidate for transplantation is made by the individual center, but if the patient (or the parents, in the case of a child needing a transplant) feels they have been unfairly evaluated, they have the right to seek a second opinion. The United Network for Organ Sharing (UNOS) Patient Services Department, the organization that manages organ transplantation in the United States, can assist with this process if necessary.

If the transplant team members decide the patient is a suitable transplant candidate, his or her name will be added to the OPTN's national waiting list. The patient's "waiting time" begins at this point, which is important because the length of time on the waiting list is sometimes a consideration in allocating donor organs. OPTN policy allows candidates for organ transplant to be listed at more than one center, so individuals may choose this route if feasible given their circumstances and given considerations such as the distance to be traveled and compatibility of each center with their health insurance. However, the individual seeking to be listed must go through the evaluation process and be approved at each center to which they apply, and some centers may not accept multiple-listed patients. In addition, being listed at multiple centers served by the same organ procurement organization may not help reduce waiting time, although being listed at centers in different parts of the country may help.

Organ donation rates are higher in some areas than others, so if a person lives in an area with low donation rates, they might also choose to be listed at a center in an area with higher donation rates. Waiting time can be transferred (e.g., an individual might have 12 months of waiting time at one center and 15 months at another and can switch the times to have 15 months at the first and 12 at the second). However, waiting time cannot be added, so an individual with 15 months of waiting time at one center and 12 months at another cannot add them to claim 27 months of total waiting time.

THE MATCHING PROCESS

The national waiting list, which is actually a computerized database, is managed by OPTN. The purpose of the waiting list is to match potential donors to potential recipients, a complex process because different factors are granted different levels of importance depending on the organ to be transplanted. In the United States, the process of matching is performed by organ-specific computer algorithms within the UNet system, a national computer database maintained by UNOS. When an organ becomes available, information about each available organ is matched with information about potential recipients, and the UNet system generates a rank-ordered list of candidates to be offered each organ.

The process of matching begins by screening out anyone on the transplant waiting list who is incompatible with the donor organ. Following this initial screening process, potential recipients are ranked based on criteria determined at the national level. Some of the factors relevant to organ matching include blood type, body size, severity of medical condition, distance between the location of the donor (and their organs) and the hospital where the transplant would take place for a potential recipient, the time the recipient has been on the waiting list, and whether the recipient is immediately available for transplant. This latter requirement means that the potential recipient has been contacted and has no temporary condition, such as an infection, that would preclude the transplant from taking place immediately. Questions of distance in particular are more critical for some organs than others, depending on the length of time the organ in question can survive outside a human body. For instance, a heart or pair of lungs can only survive for 4–6 hours outside a body, while kidneys can survive for 24–36 hours. The allocation system may also work differently for people of different ages: for instance, for lung transplants, time on the waiting list is considered for recipient candidates under age 12, but not for those age 12 or older.

The matching process usually begins at the local level, with "local" in this case referring to the area served by the organ procurement organization where the donation occurs. There are 58 organ procurement organizations in the United States, and the size of the area each covers ranges from several states to just a city or part of a state. Because organs are first offered in the area where the donor was at the time of death, the fact that the matching process begins at the local level is one reason being listed at multiple transplant centers in different geographical areas may improve an individual's chances to receive a donated organ. While multiple listing is a controversial practice, some studies have indicated that this advantage is real.

If there is no suitable recipient match for an available organ at the local level, it will then be offered to people on the waiting list in a wider area. However, in some cases the boundaries of the local organ procurement organization's area may be overruled by simple proximity to the organ, if the recipient is in danger of imminent death. The feasibility of offering organs to recipients beyond the local level depends in part on how long the organ can survive outside the donor's body. Organs that can survive for longer periods outside the body, like the intestines, kidneys, liver, and pancreas are offered to candidates at the regional level (11 regions of the United States have been defined for this purpose), while the heart and lungs, which have a much shorter survival time outside a body, are offered at successively larger distances until a match is made, beginning with candidates within 500 miles of the donor site (i.e., where the donor died). If no match is made, the offer is extended to those within 1,000 miles, then to those within 1,500 miles, and finally to the organ will be offered at the national level.

For some organs, a rough match in body size between donor and recipient may be important. For instance, a recipient's rib cage must be large enough to accommodate a donated heart or lungs. Children are generally given the highest priority for receiving organs donated by other children, because children often respond better to donor organs that are similar in size to their own. Another consideration may apply to some transplants, including those of the kidneys and transplants: some recipients have a highly sensitized immune system due to previous transplants or blood transfusions, so they may be more difficult to match than a similar candidate without a sensitized immune system.

NEW ALLOCATION PROCESS FOR LIVERS (2020)

In 2020, a new system for matching liver and intestinal organs was implemented in the United States. This change had a complex history: it was originally approved by the Board of Directors of the Organ Procurement and Transplantation Network in December 2018 and was briefly implemented beginning in May 2019. However, a legal challenge to the new system meant that the previous system, based on the 58 defined donation services areas, was restored. In January 2020, a court ruling allowed the new system to be implemented once again, and it is now (as of 2021) the current system in place in the United States for the organs in question. The primary organ affected is the liver, due to the commonness of that type of transplant: almost 40,000 liver transplants were performed in the United States in 2019.

The most crucial difference in the new rules is the change in the weight granted to different priorities when allocating livers and the use of mileage rather than the geographic boundaries of the 11 transplant regions and 58 donation service areas (DSAs) in making allocation decisions. Under the new system, a donor liver will be offered first to the most medically urgent transplant candidates listed at transplant hospitals within 500 nautical miles of the donor hospital. If no suitable match is found, the liver will be offered to less medically urgent candidates within 150, 250, and 500 nautical miles of the hospital, with offers grouped by medical urgency within each distance.

The new system was developed with input from transplant and donation experts, organ recipients, donor families, and the general public. It is projected to save lives and to be more equitable, because priority for transplant is based more on medical need and less on geographic distinctions. It also gives a higher priority to potential liver recipients under the age of 18 for livers from donors younger than 18 and thus is expected to increase the number of children and adolescents receiving donor livers.

PRESERVING DONOR ORGANS

The logistics of organ transplantation are such that it may be necessary to remove a donated organ in one hospital and transport it to a different hospital where the transplant will take place. It is therefore necessary to have some way to preserve the organ, if even for a short period of time, for the period in which it has been removed from the body of the donor and not yet transplanted into the body of the recipient. Given the shortage of organs, physicians and scientists are always looking for ways to better preserve and transport donated organs so that every organ that can possibly be used for transplantation arrives at the transplant hospital in a suitable state. In addition, better methods of preservation reduce the haste with which a transplantation must take place, allowing the same surgical team to perform both the organ removal and transplantation, and lessen the need for the transplantation to be done as an emergency procedure.

The basic technique for preserving an organ outside the body is to suppress the metabolism by keeping the organ cold. In order to avoid damaging the organ while it is in this hypothermic state, the blood must be removed from the organ and replaced with a hypothermic preservation solution. This technique was pioneered in the late 1960s, when F. O. Belzer demonstrated that dog kidneys could be preserved for three days and successfully transplanted after that period, if they were constantly perfused with a liquid (i.e., the liquid was circulated to the organ similarly to the way blood is supplied to a living organ) derived from plasma and kept at a temperature of 6–8 °C (42.8–46.4 °F). Geoff Collins also demonstrated, in the same period, that kidneys could be preserved through an even simpler method: the blood was flushed out of the organ with a preservative solution and the organ kept at 4 °C, but continuous perfusion was not performed.

Many modifications of these basic systems have been used in subsequent years, with the twin goals being to increase the length of time an organ can remain viable for transplant and to improve the quality of preservation. Research initially focused on preserving kidneys, because those organs were the most commonly transplanted in the early days of organ transplantation. One thing that has changed over the years is the solutions used to preserve organs: while Collins used a solution of magnesium and phosphate, it was later discovered that the solution worked better without the magnesium. Another solution used citric acid as its chief preservative, and yet another used a solution of phosphate and buffered sucrose. When improvements in the organ transplant process, in particular the development of the antirejection drug cyclosporine, made transplant of organs such as the heart, lung, liver, and pancreas possible, different techniques had to be developed to preserve those organs as well.

In the 1980s, a team at the University of Wisconsin (UW) developed a system of cold storage that allowed livers to be preserved for two days and pancreases for three days. The solution used in this process (called the UW solution) proved to be useful for preserving a number of different organs, including the heart, lungs, and bowel as well as the liver, kidney, and pancreas. Machine perfusion, in which a perfusate (solution) is pumped through the organ mechanically, providing it with oxygen and substrates, is still used to preserve kidneys, and studies have shown that kidneys can be preserved for up to seven days in this way. Kidneys preserved in this way are also associated with a high rate of functioning immediately following transplant.

A 2018 review by Jing and colleagues noted that static cold storage (flushing the organ with a preservation solution kept at 0–4 °C and then immersing it in the solution until transplantation) remains the most common method to preserve organs for transplant. However, the same review also noted that prolonged periods of cold storage may cause tissue damage to the organ, and the cold storage procedure makes it difficult to assess organ function or to repair organs. For this reason, scientists have in some cases revived the use of perfusion, while also studying the effects of different types of solutions on organ preservation.

Hypothermic Machine Perfusion (HMP), a technique first developed in the 1960s, was revived in the 1990s as demand for organs grew and the use of Expanded Criteria Donors (ECD) expanded; ECD refers to people who might ordinarily not be accepted as organ donors, for reason such as a medical history of high blood pressure. The technique of Normothermic Machine Perfusion (NMP), in which organs are perfused at physiologic conditions (35–38 °C, similar to the normal temperature of the human body), was developed in the early 2000s and first used successfully in a clinical trial in 2011. Subnormothermic machine perfusion (SNMP), in which organs are kept in the 20–34 °C range, has also been studied in the context of organ transplantation.

The OPTN has a set of protocols for the packaging and labeling of organs and provides an organ tracking system that is used by many hospitals, although it is not mandatory. These standards include the type of containers required to transport organs, information that must be collected and displayed on the containers, and documentation that must be supplied and included with the organ being transported. OPTN standards also require that each hospital have a protocol for recording and verifying information about donor organs before they are transported.

TRANSPLANTING DONOR ORGANS

If the organ donor dies in one location and the matched transplant recipient is in another, as is often the case, the organ(s) in question must be transported as efficiently as possible from one location to another. This is a delicate process, since the time any organ can be preserved outside the body is limited and specific conditions are required to keep an organ viable for transplant. Changes in the way organs are allocated, which prioritize factors other than physical proximity, make the need for efficient transport even more necessary. Other changes in the physical environment, such as an increase in extreme weather events due to climate change, may further complicate the picture.

A 2019 report by Lara C. Pullen highlights three key challenges in transplanting organs for transplant. The first challenge is that of capacity. Often organs are transplanted by air, and most often, this means using commercial aviation flights. If a donor dies in the middle of the night, this poses a problem because few if any commercial flights are available at that time. This problem may be compounded when other factors, such as the vast reduction of commercial flights during the 2020 coronavirus (COVID-19) pandemic, mean that only a reduced number of flights are available each day. Sometimes private air flights are used, but this process is extremely expensive and also subject to problems of availability in terms of both appropriate pilots and airplanes. Typically, a number of specialists from the transplant team, including surgeons, perfusionists, coordinators, and trainees, must travel as well, which only complicates the process of providing efficient and timely transportation.

A second key challenge is that of safety. Transplant teams have died in plane crashes, and in fact, the air travel fatality rate for organ transplant teams was determined by the National Transportation Safety Board to be 1,000 higher than that of commercial airline travelers. While it is well known that traveling in a small private plane is riskier than covering the same mileage on a large commercial aircraft, this danger is compounded in the case of the transportation of organs and transplant teams because the flights are typically unscheduled and need to happen soon after an organ becomes available, which may mean flying in difficult weather or in the middle of the night. The risks involved in unscheduled travel on noncommercial flights mean that transplant surgeons might need to risk their lives in order to carry out their jobs.

The third challenge highlighted by Pullen is that of cost. Organ transplantation is already a huge costly enterprise, and the use of air travel raises costs by an estimated average of $20,000 over using ground travel. Air travel poses a particular problem if a donor has died in a location far from a major airport, and it also imposes huge costs on transplant centers and transplant recipients. Medicare reimburses only some of the cost of air transportation, while private health insurance generally does not reimburse any of it, yet someone must pay the bill. One proposed solution to this dilemma is the use of drones to deliver organs, a process that has been tested on a trial basis. In April 2019, a donor kidney was safety transported by drone to the University of Maryland Medical Center in Baltimore, where it was successfully transplanted into a patient. While this is a promising result, whether this type of solution will become viable on a more widespread basis remains to be seen.

KEY ORGAN DONATION ORGANIZATIONS

In the United States, organ donation and transplantation is managed by UNOS, which administers the Organ Donation and Transplantation Network (OPTN), under contract to the federal government. UNOS is a private, nonprofit organization established in 1984 by the order of the U.S. Congress, and in 1986, it received its first contract to manage organ donation and transplantation in the United States. For administrative purposes, UNOS and the OPTN divide the United States into 11 geographic regions, and 58 Organ Procurement Organizations (OPOs) work within the UNOS/ OPTN network.

UNOS manages the national transplant waiting list, matching donors and recipients according to policies developed in conjunction with community members and the OPTN Board of Directors. It also maintains the UNet database for organ transplant data, provides support to the transplant community, provides education to transplant professionals, provides assistance to patients and family members, and educates the public about organ donation. Each OPO has a DSA, within which they are responsible for recovering organs from deceased donors. A given OPO is the only organization in their DSA that can procure organs and is responsible for every donor hospital within the DSA. The OPO works directly with the donor's family during the end of life period and enters information into the UNet system when permission for a transplant has been obtained. The OPO also facilitates recovery of the donor organs and their delivery to the designated transplant center.

In Canada, organ and tissue donation is managed through Canadian Blood Services, a not-for-profit charitable organization funded by provincial and territorial governments but operating independently from them. Canadian Blood Services was created in 1998 and is part of the Canadian network of health care systems; it operates the national transplant registry for interprovincial organ sharing and related programs, while registration for organ and tissue donation is handled on a provincial basis. Besides organ and tissue donation and transplant, Canadian Blood Services provides blood, blood products, and transfusion and stem cell registry services for all provincial and territorial governments except Quebec; in that province, those services are provided by Héma-Québec. Another organization, the Canadian National Transplant Research Program, is a national network focused on developing new knowledge and health care practices to improve the outcomes of transplants and increase the number of organs available for transplant.

In the European Union, the legal framework for organ transplantation is contained in the European Organs Directive (Directive 2010/53/EU). This document covers all stages of the process from donation through testing, handling, and distribution and specifies quality and safety standards for organs. The European Commission collaborates with other expert bodies, including the European Centre for Disease Prevention and Control and the Council of Europe, and holds regular meeting with the National Competent Authorities in charge of implementing EU requirements. Member States within the EU may have one or several competent authorities designated to govern organ donation and transplantation within that country— for instance, in Hungary, this responsibility is shared among the Hungarian National Blood Transfusion Service, the National Public Health and Medical Officer Service, the National Centre for Patient's Rights and Documentation, and Eurotransplant International.

In Australia, organ and tissue donation is managed by the Organ and Tissue Authority (OTA), an independent statutory agency operating under the guidelines of the *Australian Organ and Tissue Donation and Transplantation Authority Act 2008*. The OTA was created as part of an effort by the Australian government to create a best practices approach to coordinating organ and tissue donation and to increase donation rates through improving community awareness and raising the capacity of the health care system. Within each state or territory, donation specialist agencies are responsible for managing organ and tissue donor activities and working with hospitals to provide professional donation services. Australia also takes part in the Australian and New Zealand Paired Kidney Exchange Program, which facilitates living kidney transplants.

Organ transplantation is one of the marvels of the modern medical system, a process that literally saves lives on a regular basis. However, the process of donation, matching, and transplantation is complex, and successful completion of this lifesaving procedure requires that many different steps along the way be precisely carried out. Among other things, an individual must give permission for their organs to be donated; after their death, their organs must be matched with eligible recipients, and the organs themselves must be transported to the transplant hospital and should arrive in usable condition; only then can the transplant itself must be carried out. The lifesaving potential of organ transplantation is hampered by the fact that in most countries, including the United States, the demand for organs for transplantation is far greater than the supply of suitable donor organs, so difficult decisions must be made about who gets an available organ (and by extension, who does not).

CHAPTER 4

Life after Donating or Receiving an Organ

Organ transplantation is not a simple process, and the adjustment process does not end with the transplant. Potential organ recipients need to be aware of the expected course of treatment and recovery following receipt of a donated organ and also the possibilities that something may go wrong in the process. Aftercare is also a relevant issue for living organ donors, who are becoming increasingly common, primarily as donors of livers, kidneys, and bone marrow. While one's medical care providers are the best sources for information in this regard, and while every case is different, this chapter provides an overview of general information regarding these topics.

LIVING ORGAN DONORS: AFTERCARE AND FUTURE LIFE

While most organs for transplant are recovered from deceased donors, donation from living donors is also possible in the case of a few organs and tissues, most notably the liver, kidney, and bone marrow. This type of donation has been increasing in recent years, and over 6,000 living organ donations are performed each year in the United States alone. In a living liver donation, the donor allows part of their liver to be removed and transplanted into another living person. This is possible because the liver can regenerate (regrow) within a person's body so that the partial livers in both the donor's and recipient's body will regrow to the normal size. Due to this ability of the liver to regenerate, plus the fact that a child's liver is smaller than an adult's, adult to child donations began being performed in the 1980s, while adult to adult donations were only attempted later.

About 5% of liver transplants come from living donors, and most often the donor is related or closely acquainted with the recipient. In general, the outcome for the recipient of a liver transplant from a living donor is as good or better than the outcome from a transplant from a deceased donor. However, the risks to the donor must also be considered in the case of living donation, while there are no such risks when the transplanted liver comes from a deceased donor. Mortality is rare for a living donor, but is estimated to occur once per several hundred cases, which is too high a rate to be considered inconsequential. A living liver donor must also consider risks such as bleeding and the need for a blood transfusion, as well as the dangers inherent in any surgery. Recovery time for a living donor typically lasts eight to twelve weeks, including the approximately six weeks required for the partial liver to grow to full size.

Most people have two kidneys, but can survive with only one, making it possible for a living person to donate a kidney to be transplanted into someone else. There are risks involved for the donor, however, so, as is the case with living liver donations, usually a living kidney donor is related to or knows the recipient well. In countries where it is legal to sell human organs (which does not include the United States), a person may also donate one of their kidneys in return for a cash payment or other compensation. Following donation of a kidney, a person may remain in the hospital for four to six days, although this somewhat depends on the type of surgery performed to remove the kidney. Side effects of living kidney donation may include itching, pain, and tenderness as the surgery heals, and patients are usually warned to avoid heavy lifting for six weeks following surgery. The donor will have a scar, and some people report long-term pain following donation, although this latter effect is rare.

A person can lead a normal life with a single kidney, and there is no evidence that having only one kidney increases the risk of kidney failure or lowers a person's life expectancy. However, there is some evidence that living kidney donors are at a greater risk of developing high blood pressure. Because of the danger of damaging the remaining kidney, living donors are often cautioned against taking up contact sports, but other forms of exercise are encouraged. A living donor also needs to be prepared for their possible range of emotional responses after donation, which can be either positive (e.g., joy, relief) or negative (e.g., anxiety, depression). The donor may need time to process his or her thoughts and feelings and may want to seek out a therapist to help work though them; often such services are available through the hospital performing the transplant, and the hospital may also be able to refer the donor to a support group.

The donor may also be concerned about the financial consequences of donation, due to increased medical care needed, missed time at work, travel expenses, or worries that health insurance will become more expensive or become unavailable. Theoretically, the latter should not occur in the United States, as the *Affordable Care Act* prohibits charging a person more or refusing coverage due to a preexisting condition, but that doesn't mean it never happens in practice. Postoperative care is usually paid by Medicare or the donor's health insurance, but other expenses, such as travel and lost wages, are typically not included. While it is important that a living donor be aware of possible negative consequences of donation, it should also be noted that most living donors (80–97%, depending on the study) rate their overall experience as positive, few report serious psychological consequences, and almost none regret the decision to become a living donor.

Bone marrow donation is used to obtain bone marrow stem cells, which are used in the treatment of some types of cancer, including leukemia and lymphoma. Sometimes surgery is required to draw bone marrow stem cells directly from the bone, typically from the posterior section of the pelvic bone, while other times the stem cells can be obtained from the blood; the latter process is called peripheral blood stem cell donation. If surgery is performed, the risk factors to the donor are primarily those involved in any surgery, including the effects of being under anesthesia. Bone marrow regenerates, but it may take several weeks for this process to be complete. In the first few days following surgery, the donor may feel pain at the surgical site and may feel weak or tired. Usually, however, an individual can resume their normal activities within a few days and will feel fully recovered several weeks following the donation.

There are minimal risks involved in peripheral blood stem cell donation. One source of side effects may be the medication administered before the donation to increase the number of stem cells in the donor's blood: these side effects may include bone pain, muscle aches, nausea, vomiting, fatigue, and headache. The donation itself requires that a catheter be placed in a vein, a process that may cause minor side effects such as lightheadedness or chills, but these symptoms normally cease when the donation is complete.

ORGAN RECIPIENTS: HOSPITAL CARE

Persons who receive a donated organ are sometimes so happy to finally be off the waiting list that they underestimate the magnitude of the organ transplantation process, as well as the time they must allow themselves to recover from it. The length of time required for transplant surgery varies, depending on the specific characteristics of the patient as well as the organ involved, and may range from as little as two hours to as much as seven hours or longer. Some patients begin their postsurgical recovery in the intensive care unit or critical care unit, depending on their specific needs and the customary procedures at the transplant hospital. Time spent in the hospital also depends on both the individual characteristics of the recipient and the organ transplanted. For instance, kidney recipients are likely to have a shorter hospital stay (e.g., 4–5 days) following surgery, as compared to kidney, pancreas, and liver recipients (e.g., 7–10 days), and heart transplant recipients often have an even longer hospital stay—a 2018 study by Todd C. Crawford and colleagues found that an average hospital stay of 19 days was required following heart transplant. If any complications occurred during the surgery, the patient would probably need to spend a longer than average period recovering in the hospital before being discharged.

Longer than usual hospital stays are concerning because they make the transplant process more expensive and consume more resources, and being able to predict which patients are likely to have a longer than average posttransplant hospital stay aids in planning postoperative management strategies for those patients. Crawford and colleagues looked at this question with regard to individuals who underwent heart transplants in the United States between 2003 and 2012. Of the 16,723 cases they studied, the average posttransplant length of stay (PLOS) was 18 days, with a margin of error of plus or minus 21 days. They were able to create a model, based on factors known at the time of transplant, to predict a PLOS of more than 30 days and successfully validated this model on a different sample of patients. Variables found to be predictive of PLOS over 30 days included recipient age and gender, donor age and gender, duration of cold ischemia time (for the transplanted heart), and a number of health factors including presence of diabetes, history of dialysis, previous cardiac surgery, use of a ventricular assist device, and chronic steroid use before transplant. A number of other variables were tested but not found to be predictive, including donor and recipient race, body mass index, and length of time on the waiting list.

IMMUNOSUPPRESSIVE DRUGS

The human immune system is composed of a complex network of cells, organs, tissues, and proteins that collectively function as the body's defense system, recognizing foreign "invaders" such as bacteria and viruses, as opposed to cells from an individual's own body. When the immune system recognizes the presence of such "invaders," it mounts an immune response that can kill them, thus preventing disease or helping the individual recover from it. Under most circumstances, therefore, the immune system is beneficial to humans and in fact is necessary to lead a normal life. The immune system also produces antibodies to fight off these invaders, and they remain in the bloodstream so that, in some cases, if a person is exposed to the same pathogen again, the immune system can fight it off much more readily. The creation of antibodies in response to pathogens is the key idea behind immunization: an individual is exposed to a weakened pathogen and develops immunity, thereby being less likely to be sickened should they be exposed to the real pathogen.

However, the immune system poses a problem in organ transplants, because the recipient's body recognizes the transplant as foreign (because it came from a different person's body) and attacks the newly transplanted organ the same way it would a pathogen. This natural immune response was an obstacle that had to be overcome before organ transplantation could become an effective way of treating organ failure. Today, a variety of immunosuppressive drugs (also called antirejection drugs) are available that prevent a transplant recipient's body from attacking the transplanted organ. However, because these drugs work by suppressing the immune system, the transplant recipient is more vulnerable to infection and disease from the many bacteria, viruses, and other pathogens that are a normal part of our world.

Balancing these two demands—suppressing the immune system enough so that the transplanted organ is not rejected, while still leaving it strong enough to fight off disease—is a delicate process. However, as more and more people have lived for an extended period following organ transplant, the medical community has become more skilled at finding this balance.

A review article by Cher Enderby and Caesar A. Keller divides immunosuppression following organ transplantation into three phases: induction, maintenance, and treatment of rejection. The risk of rejection is highest just after a transplant has been performed, so the initial or induction phase requires the administration of high doses of drugs to the organ recipient and may involve the use of antibody therapy as well. Antibody induction is most common for patients receiving a pancreas (90.4%) and least common among those receiving a liver (31.1%). Patients must be closely monitored during the induction phase, and once released from the hospital, patients must take additional precautions to reduce the risk of infection, including frequent handwashing, avoiding people who are sick or have recently been vaccinated, staying out of crowded areas, taking immediate care of any cuts or scratches, avoiding contact with animals, and foregoing gardening. Planning for induction period depends on the specific circumstances of the organ recipient as well as the medical facts of the case—for instance, are there any children in the household? Does the family have pets? Do they live in a large city, small town, or in the country?

The maintenance phase follows the induction phase. The maintenance phase may begin six months to a year after the transplant, and the medical team will inform the patient when they are ready to move into this phage. Drug doses in the maintenance phase are lower than during the induction phase, and safety measures can also be somewhat relaxed, although the recipient should still avoid people who are ill or recently vaccinated and continue ordinary hygiene routines like frequent handwashing. While the drug regimens used during this period vary from one treatment center to another, as well as based on the specific needs of each patient, according to Enderby and Keller, the most common maintenance regimen involves a combination of tacrolimus, MMF/MPA (mycophenolate mofetil and mycophenolic acid), and prednisone.

Despite the best possible medical care, it is possible that a transplant recipient will have a rejection episode, when the body rejects the donor organ. If this occurs, the levels and/or types of medication will probably need adjustment, and the patient will temporarily be more immunosuppressed and thus particularly vulnerable to infections, meaning they will need to follow similar procedures as during the induction phase. Even if a rejection episode never occurs, transplant recipients can expect to be taking medication for the rest of their lives, so the patient needs to establish a routine so they take the prescribed drugs consistently and appropriately. They also need to be prepared to deal with some side effects and restrictions and to be ready to consult their physician when side effects occur, because some may go away with an appropriate adjustment to the patient's medicine.

An organ recipient may also use adjunctive therapies, meaning treatments or drugs meant to assist the primary treatment. For instance, antimicrobial and antiviral prophylaxis is common immediately after a transplant, when the risk of infection is the highest. Prophylaxis means the drugs are given to prevent rather than treat infection. Other therapies that may be included in a patient's regiment include electrolyte replacements, insulin, diuretics, antihypertensive medications, and statins. Because osteoporosis is common after transplantation, due to the use of corticosteroids, patients may also be instructed to take supplements of calcium, vitamin D, and bisphosphates. Lung transplant recipients may also receive azithromycin to prevent bronchiolitis obliterans syndrome.

One phenomenon that has been noted in transplant patients is that the transplanted organ may be accepted without the need for immunosuppressive drugs. The mechanism bringing about this result is not fully understood, but one theory is that the immune cells that would normally attack the transplanted organ are eliminated by a second attack of the immune system. If this is correct, it might be that the high doses of immunosuppressive drugs used immediately after a transplant prevent both the "bad" attack of the immune system on the transplanted organ and the "good" attack that eliminates those attacking cells. One approach to prevent the bad attack without also eliminating the good has been implemented at the Thomas E. Starzl Transplantation Institute of the University of Pittsburgh Medical Center. This approach involves the use of an antibody-based drug that lowers the chance of acute rejection (rejection shortly after the transplant) while increasing the chance that the body will accept the transplanted organ. This drug has been compared to a "guided missile" because it only affects the immune cells that attack the transplanted organ. As time passes since the transplant, the medical team reduces the dosage of conventional antirejection drugs, trying to find the minimum dose that will work for an individual patient.

ORGAN REJECTION

Sometimes, despite the best possible medical care and patient compliance, a transplant recipient will experience organ rejection. This rejection is actually a natural response by the body's immune system, as noted above, which normally recognizes and attacks anything it recognizes as not belonging to the patient's body. Tissue typing is used to match organs to recipients who are as similar as possible to the donor, but the process is never perfect, which explains why rare early transplant successes sometimes involve identical or monozygotic twins, who share all their genes and thus are as similar as two people can possibly be.

Three types of rejection have been identified. The first type is hyper acute rejection, which occurs immediately after transplant and is generally a result of completely unmatched antigens. Due to the preparatory work that goes into matching a recipient and organ, this type of rejection rarely occurs, but it is severe threat to health, and the transplanted organ or tissue must be removed. Hyper acute rejection is similar to a blood transfusion reaction (hemolytic transfusion reaction) that can occur when an individual receives a transfusion of the wrong blood type and his or her immune system attacks and destroys the red blood cells. Fortunately, due to careful screening before a transfusion, hemolytic transfusions reactions are rare, and due to careful matching before transplant, hyper acute rejection is also rare.

Acute rejection refers to rejection from the first week after transplant up to three months after transplant. It is a normal response to the transplant and can usually be controlled by changes in medicine or dosage. The third type of rejection is chronic rejection, which occurs after at least three months of living with the new organ and can actually happen many years after the transplant. Chronic rejection is believed to occur due to damage to the organ from the immune system, which continues to mount a response to the unfamiliar organ despite the patient taking the recommended dosage of immunosuppressive drugs. A rejected organ may simply work less well over time—for instance, someone with a donor kidney may find that they are producing less urine or someone with a heart transplant may have some of the symptoms of heart failure. The patient may also experience pain or swelling around the organ; general discomfort or feeling of illness; and flu-like symptoms such as chills, cough, body aches, nausea, and shortness of breath. Fever is rare as a sign of organ rejection, although it is possible.

Organ rejection can be diagnosed through a combination of physical examination, medical tests, and a biopsy; in fact, biopsies of a transplanted organ are often performed periodically, as this allows detection of rejection before other physical symptoms become evident. Some of the symptoms of rejection are specific to the organ in question, such as yellowed skin (jaundice) in the case of a failing transplant liver or high blood sugar in the case of a failing transplant pancreas. Various medical tests, including ultrasound, CT scans, and X-rays, may aid in the diagnosis of organ rejection. Treatment often consists of increased dosages of antirejection drugs to suppress the immune reaction; when the symptoms of rejection are no longer present, the dosages may be able to be reduced. Acute rejection alone does not mean that a transplant will fail, and often the patient can recover and continue to live with the transplanted organ. However, chronic rejection is the most common cause of organ transplant failure. If antirejection medicines are not sufficient to solve the problem, the organ may need to be removed and the patient will need a new transplanted organ.

Life Expectancy After Receiving an Organ Transplant

Two types of survival are relevant to organ transplantation: graft survival and patient survival. Graft survival refers to the transplanted organ remaining functional in the recipient's body (e.g., that a transplanted kidney continues to do the job of a kidney), while patient survival refers to the individual receiving the transplant remaining alive. A patient can receive one or more transplants of the same organ following failure of the original transplanted organ, so patient survival can be longer than graft survival. Both types of survival are important because, while increasing patient survival is the primary reason transplants are done, it is also true that the longer an individual graft continues to function correctly, the better. This is particularly true in consideration of the shortage of organs available for transplant and the arduous nature of the transplant process itself, so it is preferable for a patient to survive with a single transplant rather than requiring multiple transplants of the same organ. Another key distinction in reporting is between primary transplants (the first transplant) and repeat transplants (meaning the patient has received one or more transplants of the organ before the current transplant). A repeat transplant is also referred to as a "retransplant."

The Organ Procurement and Transplantation network (OPTN) publishes numerous reports on organ transplantation in the United States, which are freely available from the website of the U.S. Department of Health and Human Services. Information is available at the national, regional, state, and center level, and customized reports can be generated through an interface provided through the Health Resources and Services Administration (HRSA)/OPTN website. Both graft and patient survival are typically reported in one-year, three-year, and five-year increments, as is standard in some other types of medical statistics (e.g., survival following a diagnosis of cancer). Length of survival time is associated not only with the type of organ transplanted but also with characteristics of the donor and recipient.

Looking at data on transplants performed between 2008 and 2015 (the most recent period for which the relevant statistics are available), OPTN reports a one-year graft survival rate of 80.9% for primary heart-lung transplants, a 58.3% for three-year survival rate, and a 49.2% for five-year survival rate. Insufficient data were available to estimate comparable statistics for repeat heart-lung transplants. For primary heart transplants, the one-year graft survival rate was 90.5%, the three-year survival rate was 84.9%, and the five-year survival rate was 77.7%; for repeat heart transplants, the one-year survival rate was 86.5%, the three-year survival rate was 75.5%, and the five-year survival rate was 67.8%. It can be seen, from the statistics relating to heart transplants, that the graft survival rate decreases with time, but this is not surprising since everyone who survived five years, by definition, also survived one year and three years. It can also be seen that repeat transplants have somewhat lower survival rates than primary transplants. Both patterns will be observed across a number of organs.

For kidney transplants, the graft survival rate for primary transplants was 94.7% for one year, 87.8% for three years, and 78.6% for five years; graft survival for secondary kidney transplants over the same periods was 93.9%, 86.5%, and 77.6%, respectively. For kidney-pancreas transplants, the one-year graft survival rate for primary transplants was 95.7%, three-year survival rate was 89.5%, and five-year survival rate was 81.4%, while for repeat transplants the survival rates were 97.2%, 80.6%, and 62.1% for one, three, and five years, respectively. For pancreas primary transplants, the one-year graft survival rate was 81.8%, three-year survival rate was 71.4%, and five-year survival rate was 60.1%, while for secondary pancreas transplants, one-year survival rate was 77.7%, three-year survival rate was 65.8%, and five-year survival rate was 51.8%.

For primary liver transplants, the one-year graft survival rate was 89.6%, three-year survival was 80.8%, and five-year survival was 61.8%; for secondary liver transplants, the corresponding one-, three-, and five-year rates for graft survival were 78.6%, 67.8%, and 61.8%, respectively. For lung transplants, one-year graft transplant survival rates were 87.2%, three-year survival rate was 68.7%, and five-year survival rate was 53.4%. Graft survival rates for secondary lung transplants were 76.0% for one year, 68.7% for three years, and 32.9% for five years. For primary intestine transplants, the one-year graft survival rate was 77.2%, three-year survival rate 60.9%, and five-year survival rate was 50.6%, while for repeat transplants, the corresponding survival rates were 67.2%, 49.0%, and 40.8%, respectively. While patient survival and graft survival can diverge over longer periods of time (a person could conceivably receive three or more transplants), for the periods covered by these statistics, patient survival after one graft is generally comparable to graft survival for a primary transplant, while patient survival after two grafts is generally comparable to graft survival of a repeat transplant; for instance for kidney transplants, the most common type of organ transplant, patient survival is identical to graft survival over one, three, and five years.

FACTORS ASSOCIATED WITH INCREASED SURVIVAL TIME FOLLOWING ORGAN TRANSPLANT

Researchers have studied which factors are associated with increased survival following an organ transplant. This question is of interest because there are more people waiting for organs than there are organs available for transplant, so one factor considered in allocating organs may be which patients are most likely to survive, and for how long, following transplantation. A study by Arman Killic and colleagues at The Johns Hopkins

Hospital found that while about half of patients who received a transplanted heart lived 10 years or more following the transplant, the probability of living that length of time was not equal for all recipients. The research team found that heart transplant recipients age 55 and younger had a 24% greater chance of survival for 10 years or more, as compared to persons older than 55. Specific age was also related to survival, with a 10% increase in survival for a decade or longer for every 10 years younger the patient was. Another factor associated with increased probability of surviving for 10 years or more was receiving the transplant at a high-volume transplant center, defined as a center that performed 9 or more heart transplants annually. Patients transplanted at the high-volume transplant centers were 31% more likely to survive for 10 years or more, as compared with those transplanted at lower-volume centers.

The Johns Hopkins team found that race was also associated with increased survival: white patients were 35% more likely to survive for a decade or longer, as compared to minority patients. General health was another factor related to survival: for instance, patients on ventilators at the time of their transplants were 47% more likely to die within 10 years following the transplant than patients not on ventilators, and persons with diabetes were one-third more likely to die within 10 years than persons who did not have diabetes. Finally, reduction in ischemic time, or the time the transplanted heart was out of the body while being transplanted from donor to recipient, was associated with increased long-term survival: a one-hour reduction in ischemic time was associated with an 11% increase in survival for a decade or longer.

A review article by Gabriel Thabut and Herve Mal identified a number of factors associated with survival following lung transplantation, based on the study of over 55,000 adult lung transplant patients who underwent a transplant between 1990 and 2014. They first note that median survival time following lung transplantation was 5.8 years and that this number increased over the years of the study. However, this median survival is lower than that for more other solid organ transplants, an issue that has raised questions about whether lung transplantation truly increases survival time. However, Thabut and Mal note that most lung transplant recipients do receive a significant survival benefit following transplantation and that further research is required to understand one major impediment to survival, that of chronic lung allograft dysfunction (CLAD), which develops in about half of all lung transplant recipients after five years.

Thabut and Mal found that the underlying disease that necessitated the lung transplant was strongly associated with median survival time. For instance, the median survival time for patients with cystic fibrosis

(CF) was 8.9 years, as compared to 6.7 years for patients with chronic obstructive pulmonary disease (COPD) with alpha-1 antitrypsin deficiency (AATD), 5.6 years for patients with COPD without AATD, and 4.8 years for patients with idiopathic interstitial pneumonia. However, they note that some of these relationships may be due to patient characteristics rather than the disease itself: for instance, CF patients tend to be younger, have fewer comorbidities, and are less likely to smoke as compared with patients with COPD. Gender was positively associated with survival (females survive longer), while the use of a ventilator or dialysis, as well as other comorbidities, was negatively associated with survival. Bilateral lung transplant (both lungs transplanted) was associated with longer survival time as compared with single lung transplant (media survival time of 7.3 years for bilateral lung transplant as compared to 4.6 years for single lung transplant), but this relationship was complicated by the fact that older and more frail patients were more likely to receive single lung transplants, while younger people were more likely to receive bilateral lung transplants.

Sven Pischke and colleagues looked at factors related to long-term survival (15 years or more) following liver transplantation. They compared the survival of transplant patients to an age-matched cohort of healthy people from the same country (Germany). Increased age was negatively associated with survival, with a higher mortality rate in patients above the median age (53) at the time of transplant. This result has been found in other studies as well. Increased BMI (body mass index, a measure comparing an individual's weight to their height) was also negatively associated with survival. Finally, patients for whom hepatitis B was the underlying disease had lower mortality than those with other underlying conditions.

Organ transplantation can extend a patient's life expectancy and improve their quality of life, but life after a transplant is unlikely to be exactly the same as life before. Fortunately, a great deal is now known about the usual progression from surgery to recovery to long-term survival, and medical care is constantly improving survival rates. With the increasing use of organs donated from living donors, the risks involved and expected time required to recover are also relevant for people considering this type of donation. Now that organ transplantation has become a common procedure, with expected survival times of five years or more, there is also considerable interest in identifying factors that are associated with successful transplant and a longer survival time following transplant.

CHAPTER 5

Religious and Cultural Perspectives on Organ Donation

A good understanding of how different people from different cultures view organ donation and transplantation is essential to anyone working in this field. One aspect of culture is particularly important in this regard: that of religion. Because many religions have particular beliefs about the integrity of the body and the end of life, and because the rituals performed shortly after death vary by religion, it's important to understand how different religious groups feel about organ donation. Of course, no religion is a monolith, and the specific beliefs and feelings of individuals may differ, but general knowledge about how the major religions view organ donation can help provide useful context.

According to a review article by Pierluigi Bruzzone, no major religion expressly forbids donating organs or receiving a transplanted organ from a donor, although some religious subgroups may have beliefs or customs that might restrict organ donation or transplantation in particular circumstances. Hence, it is particularly important to be aware of the nuances as well as the broad picture of how different religions regard organ donation and transplantation. Bruzzone also notes that no major religion decrees that organ donation is a duty or that a person's organs are somehow public property or a resource independent of the wishes of the individual—instead, even those religions that strongly support organ donation regard the decision to donate or not as a choice to be made by the individual in question and his or her family. Some religions favor organ transplantation from living rather than deceased donors, but this tends to be specific to particular subgroups and geographical areas. Xenotransplantation (the transplantation of organs or tissues from one species to another, for instance from an animal into a human) is not specifically banned by most religions, although there could be exceptions for organs from specific animals in some religions.

CATHOLICISM AND ORTHODOX CATHOLICISM

The Catholic Church, the largest Christian denomination globally in terms of number of members, encourages organ donation as an act of selfless charity. The Church's catechism (a summary of Catholic doctrine in the form of questions and answers) speaks of organ donation as a "noble and meritorious act" that should be encouraged. In 1990, the Catholic and Protestant Churches in Germany issued a joint declaration in encouragement of organ donation. Several recent popes (the pope is the head of the Catholic Church) have spoken out in favor of organ donation and at least one pope is registered as an organ donor.

Pope Francis, who was elected to the papacy in 2005, spoke to the Italian Association for the Donation of Organs, Tissues, and Cells on April 13, 2019. In this address, he referred to organ donation as both a lifesaving procedure and a social necessity, as transplantation of a donated organ often offers the only chance for an individual to go on living. He described donation as an act of social responsibility as well as a means of looking beyond oneself and expressing one's connection with the larger society of human being. However, in the same speech, Pope Francis also specified that organ donation must be uncompensated (meaning people should not be paid for donating their organs), because selling an organ would mean treating the body as a commodity, which is contrary to Church doctrine. Pope Francis was not the first pope to speak out in favor of organ donation. Pope John Paul II (in office 1978–2005) spoke publicly in favor of organ donation and praised it as an example of Christian love in the encyclical letter *Evangelium Vitae no. 86*. His successor, Pope Benedict XVI (in office 2005–2013), publicly stated that he was registered to donate his organs after death and always carried his organ donor card with him.

The Eastern Orthodox Church (Orthodox Catholic Church), the second largest Christian denomination globally, is made up of a number of autonomous denominations following several different liturgical traditions, so making any general statement about attitudes toward organ donation must be tempered by this understanding. However, leaders of several of the individual Orthodox denominations have spoken out in terms of support for organ donation and transplantation, and in 2005, the Archbishop of Athens and All Greece revealed that he had signed an organ donor card.

The Orthodox Church values the sanctity of the body and emphasizes that full respect for the bodies and souls of both the organ donor and recipient must be a primary focus when organ donation and transplantation are considered. Explicit consent must be given for donation after death (i.e., an opt-in rather than opt-out system should be used); however, the consent of relatives to donate a deceased person's organs may also be acceptable if it is not contrary to the donor's wishes. The individual donating his or her organs must freely decide to do so, without coercion or promise of payment (monetary or otherwise), and the promise to donate cannot be a reason to withdraw potentially lifesaving care. If a living donation is being considered, carrying out the donation must not endanger the life or health of the donor. From the point of view of the recipient, the transplant must be performed to improve the well-being of the recipient, and not for any experimental purpose.

The Orthodox Church's emphasis on the explicit consent of the donor has brought it in conflict with the Russian medical system, which operates under an opt-out system (organs may be removed for transplantation from a dead person unless that person has explicitly stated they do not wish to donate their organs). This conflict was highlighted in a case that received widespread publicity, that of Alina Sablina and her mother Yelena Sablina. Alina Sablina was killed while crossing a street in Moscow, and Yelena Sablina's grief at her daughter's death was compounded when she learned that multiple organs had been removed from her daughter's body before burial, including part of her lungs as well as her heart and kidneys. Yelena Sablina sought justice through the Russian court system, but lost her case, and then her appeal. The Russian Constitutional Court, in reference to this case, affirmed that Russian medical institutions were not legally obligated to notify relatives or seek their consent before removing organs from deceased individuals. In response, officials from the Russian Orthodox Church suggested that Russia change to an opt-in system. Others noted that Russia performs very few organ transplants relative to the size of its population, so the opt-out system does not seem to be performing its presumed purpose of saving lives by increasing the number of donor organs actually transplanted into people who need them.

OTHER CHRISTIAN DENOMINATIONS

There are many Protestant churches, each with their own interpretations and beliefs. For this reason, it is more difficult to generalize about Protestant attitudes toward organ donation and transplantation except to say that many churches allow and encourage both practices—donation as an act of charity and transplantation as a means to save a life. Specific beliefs and doctrines of a denomination can also change over times, as is the case with the Jehovah's Witnesses. Organ transplantation was explicitly prohibited for Jehovah's Witnesses until a few decades ago, but today the choice to donate organs or receive a transplant is considered an individual matter. Notably, Jehovah's Witnesses do not accept blood transfusions, and individual members of this religion often carry a card attesting to this fact and make their desires explicit before undergoing medical procedures. The refusal of blood transfusions is more relevant to receiving than to donating organs, as the transplantation process must be performed on a bloodless basis. There has been some controversy over placing Jehovah's Witnesses on organ waiting lists, since a member of that faith will not accept a blood transfusion even if it were the only means to save their life. Given the shortage of organs for transplantation, everyone wishes each transplantation to have the highest possible chance for success. However, procedures have been developed to increase the probability of success in a bloodless transplant operation, and successful organ transplants have been performed on Jehovah's Witnesses.

The Church of Jesus Christ of Latter-day Saints (informally known as the Mormons) does not have an official point of view regarding organ donation, although it does specify that donation should be performed for the benefit of others rather than for personal gain, so selling organs is not acceptable. Apart from that specific stricture, decisions about donating organs are considered a private matter for the individual and his or her family. The church does recommend that individuals concerning donation consult with their family and spiritual advisers and that the decision should result in a state of peace for the donating individual. Numerous other Protestant denominations do not have an official position on organ donation and leave the decision to donate or not to the individual and/ or his or her family. Churches adopting this stance include the Church of Christ, Scientist (Christian Scientists), The Society of Friends (Quakers), and the Mennonite Church.

Some Protestant denominations encourage organ donation, while still affirming that the decision to donate must be a voluntary one of the donating individual and his or her family. For instance, the Unitarian Universalist Church considers organ donation a selfless act of giving, and the choice to donate or not is left to the individual because the Church believes that people should be allowed to make decisions concerning their own body. The Southern Baptist Convention considers organ donation to be a personal matter, but the Convention has also issued declarations in support of organ donation and the possibilities it offers for saving lives. Members of the Baha'í faith are free to donate their organs after death, and some Baha'í teachings describe organ donation as a noble act and a way to be of service even after death.

The Church of the Nazarene considers donation an individual decision, but encourages those who wish to donate their organs after death to create living wills and trust to ensure that their wishes will be honored. The Church of the Nazarene has also stated that it is important that the organs available for transplantation are distributed in a moral and ethical manner to those who need them. The Episcopal Church encourages its members to consider donating organs after death and, if they decide to do so, to communicate that decision to their family. The Anglican Church has issued public support for organ donation, while recognizing that different individuals might feel differently about the process. The Methodist Church considers organ donation to be an act of charity and has stated that the chance to save a life outweighs any interference this may cause in the process of preparing a body for burial.

The Seventh-day Adventist Church does not have an official doctrine regarding organ donation and emphasizes that life and death decisions are best made by individuals and their families. However, the Loma Linda University Medical Center, which is a Seventh-day Adventist institution, carries out many organ transplants, offering some indication of the Church's support of the process. The United Church of Christ supports organ donation, although there is no statement from the General Synod on this subject because it is considered noncontroversial. The United Methodist Church has spoken out in favor of organ and tissue donation and encourages its members to sign up to be organ donors.

The African Methodist Episcopal churches (AME and AME ZION) regard donation of organs and tissues as an act of love and charity and encourage members to become organ donors. The Assemblies of God, the larger Pentecostal denomination in the world, supports organ donation as a means to save lives and because they believe that a deceased person has no further need of his or her mortal body. At the same time, according to The Assemblies of God, organ donation must be entirely voluntary, and the church urges persons considering donating their organs to reflect on the matter before making their decision and to discuss their plans with their family.

The Church of the Brethren supports educating church members about organ donation and encourages individuals to discuss the possible donation of their organs and tissues after death with their families and religious leaders. They support members signing and carrying a Universal Organ

Donor Card and including their wishes regarding donation within an advanced medical directive. They also note that the gift of donated organs must be made freely and with consideration and that it is not acceptable to hasten someone's death in order to harvest organs or for an individual to make a living donation if doing so would harm their own bodily integrity. The Disciples of Christ (also known as The Christian Church or D.O.C.) encourages organ and tissue donation among their members, stating that organ donation is an instance of sharing. In 1985, the organization passed a formal declaration encouraging members to register as organ donors and to support those who have undergone an organ transplant.

The Evangelical Lutheran Church, the largest Lutheran denomination in the United States, encourages organ donation, including both living donations and donation after death. This church regards the donation of organs and tissues as an expression of love as well as a means to contribute to another's well-being and encourages those who want to be organ donors to communicate their desires to their family and physician and to make the necessary legal arrangements including signing an organ donor card. They also encourage religious leaders to educate themselves regarding organ donation, to be prepared to counsel people seeking guidance on this matter, and churches and other religious organizations to sponsor educational programs on organ donation. However, this church has spoken out against the exchange of money for human organs, as well as any coercion to try to make someone consent to organ donation, and is in favor of assuring that the distribution of transplantable organs and tissues is done fairly and efficiently.

JUDAISM

Traditionally, the Jewish faith has placed great importance on the complete and rapid burial of a body following death and prohibits any interference with a dead body. Today, however, many Jewish authorities today believe that the ability to save lives is more important than almost any other consideration, and most branches of Judaism allow organ donation and transplantation. However, the process of organ donation is complicated by the requirement that the donor should be dead according to Jewish law before the organs are removed. The definition of when a person is truly dead is a matter of some controversy within Judaism, as some Jewish scholars believe that brain stem death is sufficient for a person to be declared dead, while others require cardiac death. For this reason, organ donation cards issued by the Halachic Organ Donor Society (a Jewish organization founded in 2001 to encourage organ donation) allow the individual to specify which definition of death they embrace.

The modern country of Israel, which regards itself as a Jewish and Democratic state, was not slow to participate in organ transplantation. The first organ transplant in Israel was performed in 1964 and involved the transplantation of a kidney from a living donor to a related recipient; the first transplantation of a kidney from a deceased donor occurred in 1965. Since 1994, organ donation and allocation has been handled on a national level, with six medical centers performing organ transplantations. However, organ donation rates have historically been low among Israelis, due in part to the tradition of not interfering with a body after death. In an effort to reduce "free riding" (taking advantage of a system without contributing to it), in 2008 Israel passed an Organ Transplant Law that gave priority for organ transplantation to individuals who have been living organ donors, have been listed for at least three years as a deceased donor, or have a first-degree relative who has been an organ donor.

For some years, organ donation in Israel may have been discouraged by the fact that Israeli citizens had easier access to organs from living donors than residents of other countries, due to Israel's geographic location and because "transplant tourism" (travel to another country in order to receive an organ transplant) was subsidized by Israeli health insurers. The combined result of access to living donation through transplant tourism and the general dislike of removing organs after death resulted, in the early 2000s, in more kidney transplants being performed on Israelis in other countries than in Israel. However, in 2008, the Israeli Parliament banned participation in organ trafficking in any country and barred reimbursement of organ transplantation services abroad involving traded or illegally procured organs. Israeli laws have also reduced the financial disincentives faced by living donors, by increasing the reimbursement for lost income and for expenses involved in the donation process. As a result of these measures, the percentage of people registered as organ donors has increased, although they remain below the rates seen in many European countries.

ISLAM

Islam is the world's second-largest religion, in terms of number of followers, and not surprisingly, there is no unanimity of opinion regarding organ donation within this faith. Over 100 edicts (*fatwas*) have been issued on organ donation, providing guidance about organ donation in the context of Islamic law. As is the case with several other religions, Islam places value on two things that may come into conflict in the context of organ donation: protecting the human body from violation and performing

60   **ORGAN DONATION**

altruistic acts that save lives. The balance found between these two competing demands has generally embraced the principle that "necessity overrides prohibition," and Islamic authorities in multiple countries have approved organ donation as an act of merit.

Muslim burial customs can conflict with the needs of organ donation, because bodies are normally buried within 24 hours of death, and a lengthy process to remove organs could conflict with this expectation. The concept of brain stem death is not embraced by all Muslims, resulting in another potential clash between the modern organ donation system and religious views. Even when organ donation is supported by Islamic doctrine, the choice to donate is left to the individual, as it is in other religions. Historically, Muslims have been reluctant to participate in the organ donation process, resulting in low numbers of individuals registered as organ donors in many Muslim countries. Many Muslims are also reluctant to receive transplanted organs from a cadaver (dead body), and thus, organs from living donors constitute the majority of transplants taking place in some Muslim countries.

BUDDHISM AND HINDUISM

The classification of a number of somewhat related religious practices under the term "Hinduism" is a product of 19th-century British scholarship rather than a label chosen by those so classified, and unlike many Western religions, Hinduism has no central religious authority. However, the term "Hindu" is in common use today to describe the faith of some one billion people, who share some rituals, practices, and texts in common, while also differing in other specific aspects of their beliefs and practices. According to the Hindu Temple Society of North America, the decision to donate one's organs is a choice made by an individual, and there is no prohibition against organ donation in any Hindu law. Hindu scholars have also spoken in favor of organ donation, and a spokesperson for the World Council of Hindus has stated that sustaining life through organ donation is an example of righteous living (*Dharma*).

The concept of transplanting body parts from one person or animal to another is featured in several stories in Hindu mythology. For instance, Ganesha, a deity worshipped by many Hindus, is commonly portrayed as having the body of a man and the head of an elephant. Several different stories explain how he came to take this form, including one in which the god Shiva beheaded a human child and then replaced his head with that of an elephant. Hindu scriptures include passages that can be interpreted as supporting organ donation, and organ and limb transplantation are mentioned in the Vedas, a body of ancient religious texts sacred to Hinduism. Although belief in the transmigration of the soul and in reincarnation is part of Hinduism, there is no belief that physical integrity of the body is necessary for these processes to take place. As stated by one scholar, the donation of an eye in this life does not mean the person will be lacking an eye in the next.

Buddhism has no official doctrine for or against organ donation and considers the choice to donate or not to be a matter of individual conscience. Buddhist scholars differ on the question of organ donation, due in part to traditional beliefs about the death process (which continues after what Western physicians would consider physical death). The death process is an important part of Buddhist life, but maintaining the integrity of the physical body per se is not crucial. However, some Buddhists believe that the spiritual consciousness remains in the body for days after a person has stopped breathing and that death does not occur until this spiritual consciousness has left the body. This interpretation of death poses an obvious problem for organ donation.

However, Buddhism also places a high value on compassion, and because donating one's organs could save another person's life, organ donation is recognized as a compassionate act. Buddhism states that the choice to donate must be made freely (i.e., it must truly be the wish of the person making the decision), and the care of a person near death should never be compromised in the attempt to save another's life. It is also considered essential that a potential donor should discuss his or her plans with family members.

OTHER RELIGIONS AND CULTURES

Sikhism, a religion founded in the 15th century, emphasizes the importance of performing selfless service and putting the needs of others above those of yourself. There are no strictures against organ donation in Sikhism, and the practice is generally highly regarded as an example of a noble act performed to save the life of another. Sikhs believe in a continuous cycle of rebirth, but it is not necessary to have a physically intact body in order to take part in this process. Instead, the soul is considered to be the immortal part of a person, while the body is simply a vessel that is left behind and is dissolved through natural processes. Many Sikh leaders and scholars have spoken of organ donation as one of the greatest gifts one person can give to another.

Shinto is a Japanese belief system, although there is debate about whether or not it should be considered a religion. Shinto has no central authority and is primarily observed by people in Japan and by persons of Japanese descent. Being an observer of Shinto does not conflict with participation in other religious traditions, and many Japanese people take part in some Shinto rites or customs alongside other religious practices. The influence of Shinto on Japanese attitudes toward organ donation is therefore relevant, even if it is not a religion in the same way as, say, Christianity or Islam.

Purity is an important concept in Shinto, and it is believed that the dead body is both impure and dangerous, so interfering with a dead body could bring about bad luck. There is also a belief that a relationship can exist between a dead person and those who had close relationships with them and that consent to donation could interfere with this process. These beliefs created a sort of cultural taboo against organ donation in Japan for many years. In fact, deceased organ donation was illegal in Japan as late as the 1990s, and people needing an organ transplant had to travel abroad for that purpose. Although the law prohibiting organ transplant from deceased donors has since been changed, strict rules regarding brain death, and the requirement of written permission from both the donor and his or her family, have also acted to discourage organ donation in practice in Japan. The percentage of Japanese who are registered as organ donors is quite low compared to Western nations, as are the number of organs transplanted. In 2017, for instance, the organ donation rate was only 0.7 per million deaths in Japan, as compared to 26 per million in the United States. In contrast to the low rates of organ donation from deceased donors in Japan, living donations are more common, and, in the early 21st century, nearly all kidney transplants performed in Japan used an organ from a live donor.

Taoism (sometimes written Daoism) is sometimes regarded as a philosophy, sometimes as a religion. However, because it is an influential force in some Asian cultures, particularly in China, it is relevant to a discussion of organ donation. The word "Tao" translates as "path," and people following Taoism emphasize following the flow of nature. Modern Taoist scholars emphasize that Taoism does not prohibit organ donation and believe that changing the body, as by donating or receiving organs, does not change the essence of life. Confucianism, which can also be regarded as either a religion or a philosophy, is also influential in some Asian countries. Filial piety is highly regarded in Confucianism, and the body is considered a gift from one's parents. Some scholars interpret this line of thought as prohibiting organ donation, but others find support for organ donation in Confucius's emphasis on the importance of righteous behavior and on giving of oneself to sustain others.

Different religions and cultures have different beliefs regarding organ donation, and it is wise for people working in the field of organ donation and transplantation to have some knowledge of these differences. This is particularly true for those involved in providing counseling to people considering organ donation, although of course there often are differences in belief and custom within each religion or culture. In addition, each person is an individual, and the decision to participate in organ donation or receipt of donated organs rests ultimately with the affected individual and his or her family. Nevertheless, knowledge of the religious and cultural beliefs of the donor and his or her family are one important part of understanding how they may feel about the donation process, and thus, anyone who works in this field needs to have a good understanding of how organ donation and transplantation is viewed in different religions and cultures.

CHAPTER 6

Alternatives to Human Organ Donation and Transplantation

The medical science of human organ transplantation is highly developed, and transplant centers and hospitals around the world regularly perform lifesaving organ transplants. However, there is a crucial limitation that prevents even more lives from being saved: a lack of organs suitable for transplant. Various methods have been tried to reduce the gap between the number of organs needed and the number available, including campaigns to encourage people to sign up as donors, changes in the requirements for organs to be considered suitable for transplant, and changing from an "opt-in" to an "opt-out" system of donation. A complementary approach to the shortage of transplantable organs is to use other methods to supplement or replace the function of a failing organ. Examples of these types of complementary approaches include the use of a life support system that can do some of the work of the organ, xenotransplantation (transplantation of organs or tissues between species), the creation of artificial organs to replace those that have failed, and the production of new organs through organ bioprinting.

SUPPORT FOR THE KIDNEYS

One of the first mechanical systems developed to treat people suffering from organ failure was dialysis, which aids people whose kidneys are not working properly. Dialysis has three main purposes: to remove excess water, salt, and impurities from the blood; to keep safe levels of chemicals such as potassium in the blood; and to help control blood pressure. Kidney failure today is classified in five stages, based on the percentage of normal kidney function remaining, from stage 1 (kidney damage but normal function) to stage 5 (kidney failure, with less than 15% of normal function). Diagnosis of kidney failure may combine several pieces of information, including the results of a test for the presence of albumin (a protein) or blood in the urine, imaging tests (e.g., an ultrasound or CT scan), and/or a biopsy; a patient's age, gender, and other factors are also relevant to the diagnosis.

Illness and death from kidney failure has been recognized since at least the time of the Roman Empire, and various treatments were prescribed in the past for kidney failure, including bloodletting, sweating, and enemas. The modern technique of kidney dialysis was developed by adapting the techniques of osmosis and dialysis used in chemical laboratories, where these techniques are used to separate substances or remove the water from a solution. Chemist Thomas Graham suggested, in the 19th century, that dialysis might be useful in medicine, and other scientists conducted animal research in the early 20th century that involved passing an animal's blood through semipermeable membranes.

The first successful dialysis treatment was developed by the Dutch physician Willem Kolff. The treatment involved running the patient's blood through a series of cellophane tubes immersed in an electrolyte solution within a rotating drum. This process removed toxins from the blood, which was then returned to the patient's body. Kolff's first patient, who was suffering from acute kidney failure, was so aided by this treatment that he was able to leave the hospital one week later. Kolff's design was improved at Peter Bent Brigham Hospital in Boston, and the resulting dialysis machine became known as the Kolff-Brigham artificial kidney.

Other physicians and scientists made important contributions to improve the dialysis process. Swedish scientist Nils Alwall described a design for a dialyzer that reinforced the cellophane membranes with metal grates and allowed control of the pressure within the dialysis machine. In 1960, American physician Belding Scribner developed a shunt that provided easier access to a patient's circulatory system, allowing for long-term treatment of renal failure with dialysis. The first patient who survived for an extended period with chronic renal failure was Clyde Shields, who lived for 11 years while receiving dialysis (he ultimately died of heart disease).

In the United States, about one-third of the adult population is estimated to have chronic kidney disease, and kidney disease is the ninth leading cause of death nationally. In 2016, over 700,000 Americans were living with kidney failure, and over 500,000 of them received dialysis treatments, with two types of dialysis in common use. In hemodialysis, the individual's blood is pumped through a dialysis machine, which removes impurities, and then restored to the individual's body. This type of dialysis is performed three or four times a week, either in a dialysis center or in the patient's home. In peritoneal dialysis, the blood is cleansed while inside the patient's body, using a special fluid; this type of dialysis can be performed in many settings, including at work or at school. Although dialysis is a lifesaving procedure, many patients find it burdensome and would prefer to receive a kidney transplant. As a result, many patients receiving dialysis are also registered on a waiting list to receive a kidney transplant, with dialysis keeping them alive while they wait for a suitable organ to become available.

Support for the Lungs

Several technologies have been developed to support or replace lung function. The iron lung, a mechanical respirator, encloses most of the patient's body, except for the head, in a metal cylinder and uses mechanically induced changes in the air pressure within the cylinder to simulate breathing. An iron lung is thus a negative pressure ventilator and simulates the normal process of breathing for people who cannot control the muscles necessary to breathe on their own. While use of the iron lung has saved many people's lives, it has the disadvantage of requiring the patient to remain inside the machine for much or all of each day, which could be claustrophobic for the patient, and which also makes it difficult to deliver other medical care.

Prototypes of the iron lung were built in the 19th century, but the first model to be used widely was created in 1928 by Philip Drinker and Louis Agassiz Shaw, both professors at the Harvard School of Public Health. For this reason, the iron lung is sometimes referred to as a "Drinker respirator." Drinker and Shaw's iron lung was first used to treat a girl suffering from respiratory failure due to polio; she recovered quickly once placed in the machine. An improved version of the iron lung was created in 1931 by John Haven Emerson, whom Drinker sued for patent infringement. Emerson was able to demonstrate that Drinker's machine was not novel, and thus not patentable, and also argued that a machine with the potential to save so many lives should not be involved in a patent dispute but should be made freely available. Following the court decision in Emerson's favor, physicians and scientists in several countries made further improvements to the iron lung, including Robert Henderson in Scotland and Edward Both in Australia. Redesigns also lowered the cost of the iron lung, and they became a common piece of medical equipment in hospitals in the 1940s and 1950s, a time during which recurring epidemics of polio (infantile paralysis) resulted in many patients needing assistance with breathing. Most polio patients spent only a few weeks inside the iron lung, after which time they would have sufficiently recovered to breathe on their own. Some patients could spend a part of each day outside the iron lung, but required breathing assistance for some of the day, particularly during sleep. A few patients remained in the iron lung for years, demonstrating that this type of assisted breathing could be used on a long-term basis. The person believed to have lived the longest period in an iron lung is June Middleton, an Australian who died in 2009, having received breathing assistance from an iron lung for 60 years.

The development of an effective polio vaccine in the 1950s by Jonas Salk, and an improved vaccine in the 1960s by Albert Sabin, followed by implementation of widespread vaccination campaigns, means that polio rarely occurs outside of a few countries (as of 2020, it is endemic only in Afghanistan, Nigeria, and Pakistan). The decline of polio and the development of other means of assisting breathing have made the iron lung largely obsolete today. However, the 2020 COVID-19 pandemic renewed interest in the iron lung as an alternative to the more modern positive pressure ventilators used to treat patients who experience difficulty in breathing.

About 20% of the earth's atmosphere consists of oxygen, and for most people, this is sufficient: their lungs absorb the oxygen they need from the air an individual breathes in. However, some medical conditions prevent people from getting enough oxygen through normal breathing, including chronic obstructive pulmonary disease (COPD), pneumonia, cystic fibrosis, and asthma. People with these conditions may suffer from low levels of oxygen in their blood. This condition can be helped through oxygen therapy, in which an individual breathes in a direct supply of oxygen through a mask, breaking tube, or nasal prongs.

An individual may need supplemental oxygen for only a short period of time, or they may require it for years. The oxygen can be stored as a gas or liquid in a metal tank or supplied through an oxygen concentrator, which filters and compresses ambient air and supplies purified oxygen to the patient. Both oxygen tanks and concentrators are available in portable models that allow an individual to move about while receiving oxygen therapy. Due to fire hazard, smoking or the presence of any type of flame is not permitted near an individual receiving oxygen therapy.

Another option for those who need extra help breathing is a positive pressure ventilator. As the name suggests, this type of ventilator pushes air or some mix of gases directly into the lungs, through a tube in the mouth, nose, or windpipe (the latter requires a tracheotomy, i.e., surgery to create an opening in the windpipe). Ventilators were originally developed for use during surgery, because general anesthesia can disrupt the normal breathing process. However, they are also used for patients requiring more long-term breathing assistance and have become well known to the general public due to their use during the COVID-19 epidemic of 2020, when they provided life-sustaining support to patients unable to obtain enough oxygen through their own breathing processes. The rapid increase in patients suffering from COVID-19 led to shortages of ventilators in some parts of the world, underlining the need for an adequate supply of these lifesaving devices during outbreaks of severe respiratory illness. Positive pressure ventilators can be used for long periods, if necessary, and a variety of conditions may require their use, including pneumonia, COPD, stroke, injury to the spinal cord, and amyotrophic lateral sclerosis (ALS, also known as Lou Gehrig's Disease). As is the case with oxygen support and the iron lung, ventilators only provide life support and do not cure disease.

SUPPORT FOR THE HEART AND LUNGS

Cardiopulmonary bypass (CPB) is a method to temporarily replace the function of the heart and lungs by means of a heart-lung machine, which keeps the blood circulating and the oxygen and carbon dioxide levels appropriate in the patient's body. Because of various risks to the patient, CPB is only used for a short period of time (e.g., up to 6 hours), most commonly during surgery that requires the beating of the heart to be temporarily halted. Examples of such surgery include coronary artery bypass grafting (CABG), mitral valve replacement, and heart or heart-lung transplantation. CPB requires the administration of the anticoagulant heparin to prevent blood clots from forming during the procedure, and the anticoagulation process must be reversed after the patient is removed from the machine.

While a prototype heart-lung machine was developed in the late 19th century, it could not be put to practical use until the discovery of heparin in 1916. Animal experiments with heart-lung machines were performed as early as the 1920s, but their first use in a human patient dates from 1951. While the patient in that initial use of a heart-lung machine during surgery died, two years later, two physicians at the Thomas Jefferson University Hospital in Philadelphia performed successful heart surgery using a heart-lung machine. Today heart-lung machines are a standard piece of equipment for certain types of surgery and used during thousands of operations per year in the United States alone.

Patients who require longer-term support to their heart or lungs may receive extracorporeal membrane oxygenation (ECMO), which can be continued for several weeks, usually in the intensive care unit (ICU) of a hospital. An ECMO machine is connected to an individual through tubes inserted in their veins and arteries, which allow the machine to mimic the process of blood circulation in a healthy person. The ECMO machine pumps the patient's blood into an oxygenator (artificial lung), which removes carbon dioxide from and adds oxygen to the blood and then pumps this oxygenated blood back into the patient. Patients on ECMO must take anticoagulant medications, and the ECMO process must be supervised by a medical specialist who adjusts the machine as necessary so the patient's levels of oxygen and carbon dioxide remain appropriate.

ECMO provide life support, but does not cure the condition that made its use necessary. Often a patient remains on ECMO for just a few hours, until their body can function on its own, while others may remain connected to the machine for up to several weeks. Some people on ECMO are waiting for an organ transplant, while others are being treated for a medical event, such as a heart attack or lung infection. If a person's condition improves, the amount of support provided by the ECMO machine can gradually be reduced, and eventually, the person can be removed from the machine. However, if a person's condition does not improve, and the prospect of a heart and/or lung transplant does not seem to be forthcoming in the near future, the patient's health care providers will need to inform the patient and family and have a discussion about whether or not use of the ECMO machine should be continued.

XENOTRANSPLANTATION

For the purposes of this chapter, xenotransplantation will be defined as the transplantation of organs, tissues, or cells from a nonhuman animal source into a human being. Research into xenotransplantation is motivated in large part by the shortage of human organs suitable for transplant. While the potential for xenotransplantation is immense, because the supply of animals able to supply organs and tissues to humans is essentially unlimited, it also carries great potential risks. These include infecting a transplant recipient with a virus or other infectious agent from the animal donor, which could then be spread to other humans. Some of the most severe epidemics of the 20th and 21st centuries, including AIDS, SARS, and COVID-19, have been caused by viruses believed to have originated in animals before migrating to humans, so any procedure creating the opportunity for this type of cross-species virus migration must be regulated carefully.

The first attempts at xenotransplantation took place in the early 20th century, before any successful human-to-human organ transplants had taken place. However, none of these early transplants were successful, and xenotransplantation was temporarily abandoned. After the discovery of immunosuppressive drugs in the 1960s, interest in xenotransplantation revived, and in 1963, Dr. Thomas Starzl successfully transplanted kidneys taken from baboons into six human beings; one of the recipients survived 98 days with the transplanted kidney. Also, in the 1960s, Keith Reemtsma performed 13 operations in which both kidneys from a chimpanzee were transplanted into a human; he chose the chimpanzee as the donor based on its close evolutionary relationship to humans. Most of Reemtsma's transplants failed within one to two months, due to either rejection or infection, but one recipient lived for nine months following the transplant. James Hardy performed a chimpanzee-to-human-heart transplant in 1964, but the patient died within a few hours.

In 1983, Leonard Bailey successfully transplanted a heart from a baboon into an infant girl (known in newspaper reports as "Baby Faye"). The operation was successful, but the patient died 20 days later, possibly due to incompatibility of blood types between the donor and recipient. However, the broad publicity received by this case had the beneficial effect of helping to raise awareness of the need for infant organs for transplant. In 1993, a team headed by Carl Groth attempted to implant pig islets into human diabetic patients; although some of the islets survived, the patients did not benefit clinically. Xenotransplantation was temporarily brought to a halt in 1997, when it was banned globally due to concerns about viruses, in particular that it could provide a route for the transmission of porcine endogenous retrovirus (PERV) to humans. Since that date, further studies have found no evidence that this virus could produce infection in other species, and today research into xenotransplantation and its potential to improve human health is being carried out in numerous countries around the world.

ARTIFICIAL ORGANS

One alternative to organs from human donors is the creation of entirely artificial organs that can be transplanted into people. The most notable success in this regard is the artificial heart, and research is currently underway to produce other artificial organs for transplant into humans, including an artificial lung, kidney, and liver. Early research on the creation of an artificial heart was done on animals. In 1949, William Sewell and William Glenn implanted an artificial heart pump into a dog, and in 1957, Willem Kolff successfully implanted an artificial heart into a dog. Kolff founded an artificial organs program at the University of Utah, where one of his students, Robert Jarvik, was assigned to manage a project to create an artificial heart.

The Kolff group performed many experiments on cattle, improving each version of their artificial heart, and in December 1982, Kolff successfully transplanted the Jarvik 7 artificial heart into Barney Clark, a patient who was suffering from congestive heart failure. Clark survived for 112 days with his new heart. In November 1984, William C. DeVries performed the world's second artificial heart transplant, using the Jarvik 7 once again; the recipient was William Schroeder, who survived 620 days before dying of a lung infection. Today, over 1,300 people have received a Jarvik heart or one of its more modern equivalents, including the SynCardia temporary artificial heart. Several other models of artificial heart have also been developed. Artificial hearts are most commonly used today as a bridge to transplantation, so a person who is waiting for a heart from a human donor, but whose own heart is currently failing, may have an artificial heart implanted to keep them alive until a donated heart becomes available.

Artificial kidneys are not yet available for human use, but a research team at the University of California at San Francisco, led by Shuvo Roy and William H. Fissell, is developing an implantable artificial kidney that has been successfully used in animal trials. This device has two components: a hemofilter or blood filtration system to remove toxins from the blood by passing it through silicon membranes and a bioreactor to perform other functions of the kidneys, including maintaining fluid volume and blood pressure, producing hormones, and regulating salt levels.

A team of researchers at the Mayo Clinic created the Mayo Spheroid Reservoir Bioartificial Liver (SRBAL), a bioartificial liver that has been successfully tested in animal trials. The SRBAL functions outside the body, similar to a dialysis machine, but differs from dialysis in that it contains live hepatocytes (liver cells) of human or animal origin that perform the same work the liver normally does in the body. If animal cells are used, they come from genetically engineered pigs. The SRBAL is intended for three groups of patients: those with acute liver failure who are awaiting a donated human liver; those who have suffered temporary liver damage, for instance, due to an overdose of acetaminophen, but whose liver is expected to regenerate; and those who are suffering from liver failure but are not eligible for transplant due to reasons such as a high levels of antibodies or cancer.

ORGAN BIOPRINTING

Organ bioprinting, sometimes called 3D organ bioprinting, creates living tissues by building them up, layer by layer, from bioinks (droplets of living cells or biomaterials) deposited on a substrate. Although it uses different materials, the process of bioprinting is therefore somewhat similar to the 3D printing techniques used to create machine parts and the like (including "replacement parts" for the human body, such as heart valves and spinal disks). However, due to the complexity of human organs, the bioprinting process is much more complex, and success in creating living tissue that will function in the human body as well as the organ it is meant to replace has proven elusive. However, some components of organs have been produced in this way—for instance, a team from Carnegie Mellon University has created full-size heart components, including valves and ventricles, through bioprinting.

One key challenge in organ bioprinting is the thickness and complexity of the organs most in demand, including the heart, liver, and kidneys. These organs require vascularization, which performs tasks including supplying the tissues with oxygen, nutrients, and growth factors, as well as gas exchange and removal of waste products. In 2019, a team of scientists from Rice University announced they had created a technology called SLATE (stereolithography apparatus for tissue engineering), which enables creation of the kind of complex vasculature required in human organs. However, the process has only been demonstrated so far in parts of organs—in the case of the Rice team, air sacs that allow gas exchange in a manner similar to the way this process happens in the human lung. Other research groups are working on creating components of bioprinted livers, kidneys, and corneas.

The greatest obstacle to saving more lives through organ transplantation is the lack of sufficient donor organs. In addition to methods aimed at acquiring more organs suitable for transplant, many people are working on alternative methods to replace or support organs that are not functioning well. Examples of these alternative methods include the use of support systems such as dialysis and ECMO; development of techniques to transplant cells, tissues, and organs from animal sources (xenotransplantation); the creation of artificial organs such as the Jarvik heart; and the development of methods to creation new organs from living cells through 3D bioprinting.

PART II

Controversies and Issues

CHAPTER 7

Practical and Logistical Issues in Organ Donation and Transplantation

Organ donation can be a lifesaving treatment and in some cases is the only effective course of treatment available to an individual patient. Improvements in technology and the practice of medicine have made organ transplantation safer, and in many countries, the number of organs transplanted is increasing each year. However, in order to perform an organ transplant, you must first have a suitable organ available, and in many countries, the demand for organs far exceeds the supply. Donated organs must also be allocated to the individuals who need them and must then be transported to the recipient while remaining in a condition suitable for transplant. Different countries use different approaches to encourage people to donate their organs, to allocate those organs, and to bring the recipient and organ together so that the transplant may take place.

THE UNMET NEED FOR ORGANS

One of the greatest challenges in organ transplantation is to secure enough donor organs to meet the needs of all the patients who could benefit from receiving a transplant. The success of organ transplantation as a lifesaving method has increased the demand for organ transplants, and even as more transplants are performed each year, there is an even greater increase in the number of individuals who would benefit from a transplant. These individuals are generally placed on a waiting list, and some die before an organ becomes available. In 2020, for instance, the Organ

Procurement and Transplantation Network (OPTN) reported that 17 people in the United States died, on average, per day while waiting for an organ transplant. According to a 2017 study by Sebastian Giwa and colleagues, the number of individuals on waiting lists understates the number who could benefit from a transplant. For instance, they estimate the true need for heart transplantation at over 10 times that indicated by the number of people included on waiting lists. In addition, some researchers estimate that if there were no supply constraints to receiving an organ transplant if needed, the likelihood of an individual living to age 80 or older in the United States would double.

According to United Network for Organ Sharing (UNOS), in the United States, on average, one person is added to a transplant waiting list every nine minutes. As of October 2020, 108,597 individuals in the United States were registered on a waiting list for one or more organs; some of those individuals were listed more than once, so a total of 119,259 separate registrations for donor organs existed on U.S. waiting lists. The most common organ for which an individual was registered was for a kidney (91,754 individuals), followed by a liver (12,145 individuals), a heart (3,505 individuals), both kidney and pancreas (1,721 individuals), a lung (995 individuals), and a pancreas (890 individuals). Smaller number of people were waiting for other organs or body parts, including the intestines, uterus, and abdominal wall.

The number of individuals on a waiting list for an organ has increased over the years in the United States. Again according to UNOS, in 1995, 30,470 individuals were listed on one or more waiting lists to receive one or more organs. By 2000, this had increased to 39,282 individuals on waiting lists, to 44,535 by 2005, and to 51,812 by 2010. Numbers have continued to increase since then, with 53,048 individuals listed in 2015, 54,298 in 2016, 54,885 in 2017, 58,702 in 2018, and 61,229 in 2019. The number of listings (a different statistic, because one person could be included on multiple waiting lists) shows a similar pattern of increase over the years. In 1995, there were 33,023 individual registrations on organ waiting lists in the United States, a number that increased to 43,011 in 2000, 48,889 in 2005, 56,423 in 2020, and 57,614 in 2015. More recently, there were 58,888 registrations on organ transplant lists in the United States in 2016, 59,683 in 2017, 63,629 in 2018, and 66,784 in 2019.

Time spent on a waiting list for organ transplant and the probability of a wait-listed individual dying before receiving a transplant depend on the type of organ required, as well as other factors such as the recipient's blood type and the geographic region in which the recipient is wait-listed. Detailed information with breakdowns according to these factors is available from the UNOS website and the annual reports of the Health Resources and Service Administration, part of the U.S. Department of Health and Human Services; data for the three most common types of organ transplant will be covered here. In 2018 (the most recent year for which a report is available), 29.5% of individuals on a waiting list for a kidney had been listed for less than 1 year, 19.7% for 1 to less than 2 years, 15.1% for 2 to less than 3 years, 11.1% for 3 to less than 4 years, 8.4% for 4 to less than 5 years, and 16.3% for 5 or more years. Of the 34,591 individuals removed from the waiting list for a kidney transplant in 2018, 4,193 were removed because the patient died and 4,240 were removed because the patient became too sick to receive a transplant.

Among those individuals waiting for a liver transplant, according to the same report, 46.5% had been on the wait list for less than 1 year, 18.3% for 1 to less than 2 years, 9.7% for 2 to less than 3 years, 6.6% for 3 to less than 4 years, 5.0% for 4 to less than 5 years, and 13.9% for 5 or more years. Of the 12,267 individuals removed from a liver transplant waiting list in 2018, 1,260 were removed because the individual died, and 1,211 were removed because the patient became too sick to receive a transplant. Among those waiting for a heart transplant, 52.1% on a waiting list had been listed for less than 1 year, 21.3% for 1 to less than 2 years, 10.7% for 2 to less than 3 years, 6.2% for 3 to less than 4 years, 4.3% for 4 to less than 5 years, and 5.5% for 5 or more years. Among the 4,001 individuals removed from a waiting list for a heart transplant in 2018, 268 were removed because the patient died and 272 because the patient became too sick to receive a transplant.

The United States is not the only country experiencing a shortage of donor organs. According to the Council of Europe, an organization representing 47 member states, in 2019 over 150,000 patients in Europe were registered on organ donation lists. About 48,000 new patients are added to waiting lists each year in Council of Europe countries, on average, nearly 1 new patient every 10 minutes. Over 6,000 patients on waiting lists died in 2019 without receiving an organ, an average of about 18 such deaths per day.

OPT-IN VS OPT-OUT SYSTEMS

Most countries use one of two systems for organ donation after death. In an "opt-in" system, an individual must clearly indicate, often through completing some registration procedure, that they wish for their organs to be donated after their death. In this system, it is presumed that individuals do not wish to donate their organs after death unless they have specifically indicated that they do. In an "opt-out" system, an individual is assumed to be willing to donate their organs after death unless they have specifically indicated their wishes to the contrary, again typically by completing some official paperwork. In an opt-out system, therefore, it is presumed that an individual wishes to be an organ donor unless they have specifically indicated otherwise.

It might seem that this distinction is primarily of philosophical rather than practical importance, since in either case an individual has the same rights to indicate whether or not they wish to donate their organs after death. In an ideal world, where everyone has equal access to legal and bureaucratic procedures, and equal understanding of their meaning and implications, that might be true. However, even in this ideal world, it can be argued that the choice of one system rather than the other can have a significant influence on individual behavior, resulting in substantial differences in the number of organs available for transplantation from deceased donors. This argument is based on a substantial body of empirical research that demonstrates that most individuals do not make decisions according to the "rational man" hypothesized by classical economics, but instead are strongly influenced by changes in the wording of a question or how a response is elicited.

Behavior science research highlights the fact that context can play a strong role in influencing people's judgments and decisions. One topic of particular interest in organ donation is the influence of the default option, i.e., what option is in effect if an individual takes no action. In the case of an "opt-out" system, the default option is for a deceased individual's organs to be evaluated for transplant potential, while in the case of an "opt-in" system, the default option is for a deceased individual's organs to be assumed to not be available for transplant. Because different countries have different policies regarding organ donation, they present a natural experiment on the effect of opt-in versus opt-out policies. The difference in the proportion of organs available for transplant following death, from one country to the next, can be surprising. For instance, according to a research article by Shai Davidai and colleagues, many opt-out countries have a donation rate of 90% or more, while some opt-in countries have a rate of 15% or less.

Davidai and colleagues suggest that the differences in organ donation may have to do in part with a framing or contextual effect, in which case the meaning assigned to organ donation differs in opt-in versus opt-out systems. Their research draws on work by the social psychologist Solomon Asch, who found that people assigned different meanings to the term "rebellion" in the sentence "a little rebellion now and then is a good thing" depending on whether they were told the phrase was attributed to Thomas Jefferson or Vladimir Ilyich Lenin (cited in Davidai et al. 2012, 1502).

To clarify how treating opt in or opt out as the default changed an individual's perception of organ donation, Davidai and colleagues conducted a series of experiments. In the first pair of experiments, Americans responded to the hypothetical situation of living in an opt-in or opt-out country and were asked to identify the magnitude of the decision to donate their organs or not. Participants felt that choosing to donate one's organs after death represented a significantly more substantial action in an opt-in rather than an opt-out country, and choosing to not be an organ donor was a more substantial action in an opt-out than in an opt-in country. This suggests that a national opt-out policy might lead to a larger number of deceased organ donors, because most people are inclined to make the default choice suggested by the national policy rather than to make a choice contradicting it. To place these decisions in a more concrete context, individuals placed in the hypothetical context of living in an opt-in country saw choosing to donate their organs as similar to leaving half of one's estate to charity or taking part in a political campaign, while choosing to not donate felt more like leaving 5% of one's estate to charity or voting in an election.

Davidai and colleagues then repeated the experiment in two culturally similar countries, Germany and Austria, to find if there was an effect of actually living in an opt-in (Germany) or opt-out (Austria) country. They found that in the opt-in country (Germany) the choice to donate one's organs after death was relatively meaningful and substantial, while in the opt-out country (Austria), that same decision was found to be relatively insubstantial and lacking in meaning. To put it in more concrete terms, in Germany the decision to donate one's organs after death was found to be similar to working overtime without compensation or donating 20% of one's income to charity, while in Austria, it was found to be similar to fulfilling one's work responsibilities or donating one's income to charity.

In a third experiment, American participants rated a variety of prosocial behaviors (including organ donation) in terms of the effort or self-sacrifice they required, after thinking about the organ donation policies of two European countries, one of which (The Netherlands) had an opt-in default and one (Belgium) that had an opt-out default. As predicted, participants who thought about the opt-in country felt organ donation was more significant and meaningful than those who thought about the opt-out country. Those in the opt-in group likened organ donation to extremely prosocial acts, such as giving away half of one's wealth to charity or going on a hunger strike in support of a cause, while those in the opt-out group likened organ donation to allowing someone to take a place ahead of oneself in line or volunteering to help the poor. The result of these experiments suggests that national policies play an important role in how organ donation is viewed and that people in general consider making a choice opposite that of the national policy to be more extreme behavior, and therefore less likely to occur, than making a choice aligned with the national policy.

The participants in Davidai et al.'s studies were reacting to hypothetical situations, and of course, the decisions people make in a real context may be quite different. Adam Arshad and colleagues reported in a 2019 article the results of their examination of the actual rate of organ donation in 35 countries registered with the Organisation for Economic Co-operation and Development (OECD); of the countries in their study, 17 had opt-out policies and 18 had opt-in policies. The two groups of countries were comparable on factors such as GDP (gross domestic product, a measure of economic activity within a country, specifically the value of goods and services produced in a year in a country), tax rate as a percentage of personal income, primary religion, and health care spending; the only significant differences among the two groups were that the opt-out countries were more likely to be European (as opposed to North or South American, Asian, or Australasian) and to have a civil rather than a common law system. The results of their study suggest that a policy change from opt in to opt out is not a simple fix for the shortage of donor organs.

Arshad and colleagues found significant differences among the two groups of countries in only two comparisons: total living donors per million population (4.8 for the opt-out group, 15.7 for the opt-in group) and living kidney transplants per million population (4.5 for the opt-out group, 15.2 for the opt-in group). Living organ donation would not be affected by a country having an opt-in or opt-out system for deceased organ donation, so while this is an unexpected result, it does not address the question of how to increase organ donation after death. On factors that might be expected to differ between the two country groups, differences were sometimes observed between the two groups, but these differences were not statistically significant. Of course, the definition of statistical significance is based on conventions in medical research and is influenced by a number of factors, including sample size and variability within the groups, so it's worth looking at the descriptive results as well. In addition, it is worth keeping in mind that results comparing groups of countries do not predict what will happen in any individual country or region, and some countries and regions, such as Wales, have found that consent for organ donation increased after changing from an opt-in to opt-out policy.

Counties with an opt-out policy had, on average, a higher rate of deceased donors (20.3 per million population) than did opt-in countries

(15.4 per million), but the difference was not significant ($p = .195$). The p-value is a measure of how likely the observed results are if the two groups do not differ, and usually a p-value of 0.05 or less is required for statistical significance, meaning such results would occur by chance 5% or less if there were no differences between the groups. Deceased kidney transplantation was higher in the opt-out countries (30.3 per million) as compared to the opt-in countries (23.4 per million), but with a non-significant p-value of 0.134. When deceased and living kidney transplantation were considered together as total kidney transplantation, the opt-in countries had a higher rate (42.3 per million population versus 35.2 per million) due to their higher rate of living kidney transplantation, but again this difference was not statistically significant. Similar patterns were found for other types of transplantation. The authors also performed a multivariate analysis (using a model adjusted for a number of country-specific variables), but found only three significant differences between the groups of countries: opt-in countries had a higher rate of living donors (15.9 per million population versus 5.0 per million) and a higher rate of living kidney transplantation (15.4 per million population versus 4.6 per million), while opt-out countries had a higher rate of deceased kidney transplantation (31.0 per million population versus 21.8 per million).

METHODS TO INCREASE ORGAN DONATION

Given that a lack of suitable donor organs is a primarily limiting factor in the number of people who can receive organ transplants, various methods (besides changing from an opt-in to an opt-out policy) have been tried to increase organ donation. One obvious method, paying individuals to donate their organs, is widely considered unethical and is illegal in most countries. While black market (illegal) organ markets are believed to exist in some countries, the furtive nature of such operations makes them difficult to study, and ethical and legal concerns preclude considering the open sale and purchase of human organs as a feasible method to increase donation. Similarly, any method to coerce individuals to donate their organs (and payment is sometimes considered a form of coercion, particularly if the potential donor is poor and the payment is large compared to what they could expect to earn through working) would be universally condemned as a violation of the rights of the individual. For these reasons, altruistic donation will remain the rule in nearly all countries, and so any efforts to increase organ donation must be planned and executed within that framework.

Efforts to increase organ donation generally rely on some combination of nonmonetary incentives, simplification of the donation process, and education of potential donors and their families. An example of a non-monetary incentive is the system of paired donations used to increase the number of successful kidney donations and transplantations. In this type of a system, a living donor and recipient who are incompatible as a pair are listed on an exchange, and a system is used to match them with compatible donors and recipients. Because of the many factors involved in a successful match, often a chain of donors and recipients is necessary, each donor matched with a suitable recipient. This type of system is only useful when living donation is possible and has been used most often with kidney donations.

For donations after death, one system used in a few countries, including Israel and Singapore, is to give priority on organ waitlists to individuals who are registered as donors; sometimes first-degree relatives of those registered as donors are given priority as well, and sometimes a donor must be listed for a specific number of years before they gain priority. Although this system is not the official policy in the United States, for a few years a private club called Lifesharers operated under similar principles. Lifesharers, founded by Dave Undis as a nonprofit organization in 2002, was meant to increase organ donations and transplants. The basic concept behind the club was that those who joined the club agreed to donate their organs after death, in return receiving priority for available organs from other group members should they themselves need an organ transplant. If no one within the club needed organs available for donation, the organs could be donated to a nonmember. Some ethicists objected to the existence of Lifesharers, since it existed outside the national organ donation network (UNOS) and because allocation of available organs was not based on the principle of granting organs to those in greatest medical need of them. Lifesharers ceased operation in 2016, and it is not known how many, if any, successful organ donations and transplantations were carried out among members. In general, large networks are preferred in organ donation terms because only a small percentage of people die in circumstances that allow their organs to be used for transplantation, and the possibility of making an appropriate organ-recipient match is greater in a large rather than a small network.

Simplification of the donation process has already been achieved in many countries, so an individual can indicate their desire to be a donor when renewing their driver's license or by registering on a website. These changes have increased the number of people registered as organ donors in many states, but the percentage of adults registered as organ donors still differs widely by state and region, even comparing states and regions that have simplified the registration process. This result suggests that bureaucracy alone is not the key obstacle in getting people to be listed as organ donors. Sometimes people have a cultural or religious objection to organ donation (which must, of course, be honored) or distrust the medical system in general, but in many cases, potential donors are simply unaware of the lifesaving potential of organ donation and will consent to be registered as a donor once they become aware of that potential. Campaigns tailored to local communities are particularly important, because of the need to be sensitive to local customs and beliefs and because the decision to donate requires broaching highly charged topics such as life and death. Peer influence can also be important, and one focus of some educational campaigns is to change the expected norm from "don't donate" to "donate."

One anecdotal example of the potential positive effects of informing people about the benefits of organ donation came through the case of Nicholas Green, a seven-year-old British boy who was shot in an apparent case of mistaken identity in 1994 while his family was on vacation in Italy. Nicholas died a few days later in a hospital, and his parents, Reg and Maggie Green, decided to donate his organs. Organ donation was not common in Italy at the time but more than tripled following widespread publicity of Nicholas's story, including the fact that his organs and tissues (heart, two kidneys, liver, pancreas, and two corneas) helped save or improve the lives of seven different individuals in Italy. In 1993, the organ donation rate in Italy was 6.2 per million population, while by 2006, the donation rate had increased to 20 per million, and more than 120 locations and monuments are named after Nicholas Green. In addition, Reg Green has made regular visits to Italy to promote organ donation and has appeared on television alongside the individual whose life was saved by transplantation of Nicholas's liver.

Thomas Hugh Feeley and Shin-Il Moon conducted a meta-analysis to estimate the effectiveness of organ donation public education campaigns on attitudes and behaviors relevant to organ donation. Meta-analysis is a technique that allows the synthesis of results from many studies (written by different authors, possibly using different methods) on a topic, in order to draw broad conclusions about some topic. In the case of Feeley and Moon's review, they analyzed 16 studies (published articles, convention papers, or grant reports), covering 23 campaigns, with the primary outcome of interest being either signing up with an organ donor registry or notifying one's family about one's intention to donate. They also looked at the effectiveness of campaigns intended to influence attitudes toward organ donation.

Overall, Feeley and Moon found a significant positive effect for public education campaigns, with an increase of 5% over control groups (those who were not exposed to the public education campaign) in individuals registering to be organ donors or informing their families of their intent. They also found that campaigns targeting minority gains had a somewhat larger effect than those aimed at the general population and suggest that this difference may be due to the minority campaigns using messages tailored to the particular target audience, and/or because minority groups, on average, are less likely to be organ donors so that it was easier to make greater gains in donor registration and family notification with those groups.

ALLOCATION OF DONOR ORGANS

The process of deciding which potential recipient will be given an organ available for transplant is known as organ allocation. Because there are more people who could benefit from an organ transplant than there are donor organs available, and because the process of getting the organ to the recipient is complex and time dependent, allocation systems have been devised to deal with these issues. Allocation systems differ from one country to the next, so this discussion will focus on how the process works in the United States. No matter the system, however, it is important to remember that allocation systems operate in conditions of scarcity—there are not enough donor organs available for everyone who wants or needs one—so no system of allocation will make everyone happy. In addition, because issues of life and death are involved, people often have strong opinions as to how organs should be allocated, and there are legitimate differences of opinion concerning issues such as which criteria should be considered, and how much weight each should receive, in the allocation process. For these reasons, it is important to establish a set of rules for allocating organs and to make those rules publicly available so that the process is seen as open and legitimate. Organ allocation relies on people being willing to donate their organs, and if they feel the allocation system is biased or open to manipulation by, for instance, the rich and powerful, they may be less likely to sign up to be a donor in the first place.

In the United States, the OPTN is the national registry for organ matching; it was created in 1984 by the *National Organ Transplant Act*. The UNOS, a nonprofit organization located in Richmond, Virginia, operates the OPTN under a contract from the Health Resources and Services Administration (HRSA) of the U.S. Department of Health and Human Services. Two principles govern organ allocation as carried out by UNOS: (1) justice, meaning that fair consideration is given to the medical needs and circumstances of potential organ recipients, and (2) medical utility, meaning that practical considerations concerning organ survival times and other issues are considered in the effort to maximize successful transplantations. Individuals waiting for a donor organ are listed on the registry, along with key medical information (e.g., blood type, age). When a donor organ becomes available, a computer program screens those on the waiting list to see who among them are a potential match for the organ in question.

Because there are typically multiple matches for a given organ, other factors play a role in determining how organs are allocated to recipients. One factor is geographical proximity of organ and recipient: for donor hearts and lungs, distance from the donor hospital is a key factor, because of the shorter survival times of those organs. For other types of transplants, the donation service area or region may be considered. The size of the organ relative to the potential recipient is sometimes an issue, and in general, children have priority for organs donated by other children. The medical needs of the recipient, and the urgency of those needs, are typically considered as well, and time spent on the waiting list is also considered for some organs, including kidneys and lungs. Also, for kidney transplants, the factor of "survival benefit" was added as a consideration in 2015.

Survival benefit refers to the estimated number of years a recipient would live if they received a donor organ, versus the number of years they would live without the donor organ (i.e., if they died while on the waitlist for an organ). The purpose of including survival benefit as a factor in organ allocation is to maximize the years of life gained, so a person with more estimated years of life gained would be given priority over someone with fewer estimated years of life gained. Notably, considering survival benefit as an allocation factor may work in the opposite direction from medical urgency, because a person very near death (hence, a person with high medical urgency) may well die during the transplant process or may well have other comorbidities that would reduce their expected years of lives gained following a transplant.

Suppose an individual is estimated to survive 1 year without a transplant and 5 years with a transplant: their expected survival benefit is 5–1 = 4 years. For a different person, expected to live 2 years without a transplant and 10 years with a transplant, their expected survival benefit is 10–2 = 8 years. In extreme cases, it is possible for a transplant to produce no survival benefit, which is obviously an outcome to be avoided given the scarcity of donor organs. For instance, an individual who is allocated an organ but dies during the transplantation process receives no survival benefit, but they could be argued to receive a negative benefit, since they might have lived a bit longer had they not undergone the surgery. Similarly, someone with a very mild condition might live the same number of years within a transplant as with a transplant, so again there is no survival benefit to allocating an organ to that individual.

Some scientists believe that survival benefit should be considered in prioritizing recipients for other types of transplants (besides kidneys). For instance, Douglas E. Schaubel and colleagues argue that survival benefit should be included as a factor in allocating livers from deceased donors. They frame their argument in terms of urgency versus utility. In an urgency-based system, the individual judged most likely to die on the waiting list receives the highest priority, while in a utility-based system, the individual judged likely to gain the most benefit from the transplant receives priority. They then develop an allocation system based on survival benefit, which aims to minimize mortality while prioritizing patients based on lifetime benefit. To take the simplified case of a single liver available for transplant, when the only factor considered is mortality, the organ would be allocated to the individual who had the greatest difference between their estimated waiting list lifetime (how long they would live without the transplant) and their posttransplant lifetime (how long they would live after receiving the transplant). Using a simulation process (explained in detail in their paper), they estimate that over 2000 life years would be saved annually if donor livers were allocated on the basis of survival benefit.

Consideration of geographic location is partly a necessity in allocating organs, because each type of organ is viable for transplant for only a limited time following removal from the donor's body. Another issue is that of public education and recruitment drives, which are often organized locally with the purpose of increasing donation within the local area. Because organ donation is an altruistic act, the sense of helping someone locally may be more motivating for a potential donor than the possibility of helping someone in, say, a big city on the other side of the country. This might raise issues in convincing people to sign up to be organ donors in the first place, since many people may be more interested in helping someone in their own community or state rather than elsewhere. There is also the fear that, even with clear procedures and regulations, certain transplant centers or physicians may manipulate the system to receive more than their share of organs. This possibility again raises the problem of how to convince people to donate their organs if said organs may very likely be "whisked away" to a transplant center operating for the benefit of people in another part of the country.

However, improved methods of preservation have increased the length of time that some organs remain viable, and some people feel that, within the limits of feasibility, geographic factors should not be prioritized in organ allocation, relative to medical need. This controversy exists in part due to the belief that some people in need are much more likely to receive a donated organ than others on the wait list, based on nonmedical factors such as where each potential recipient lives. This belief has been furthered by multiple registrations by few high-profile cases that have suggested that people with greater resources, and/or who have access to physicians who know how to "play the game," have made the system fundamentally unfair.

Ashley E. Davis and colleagues examined the question of whether significant disparities in waiting time for a donor kidney exist across the 58 donor service areas (DSAs) in the United States. They found that there was indeed significant variation in waiting times, which is a violation of a federal mandate, although no suggestion is made that the differences are due to deliberate policies or manipulation of the system. Based on data in the UNOS database and the United States Renal Data System, it was found that median waiting time for standard criteria donor kidneys ranged from 0.59 to 5.17 years and from 0.41 to 4.69 years for expanded criteria donor kidneys (the latter includes kidneys from a donor over age 60 or a donor over age 50 with certain complicating factors such as a history of high blood pressure or high creatinine levels). Longer waiting times were associated with being in a DSA, in which more individuals were suffering from end-stage renal disease, there were lower procurement rates for donor kidneys, and more competition among transplant centers. They also found that the disparity in waiting time increased from 2000 to 2009 and that this disparity has not been mitigated through the use of marginal organs or living donor organs. They conclude that changes would probably be required in the kidney allocation system itself in order to make waiting times more equal across DSAs.

One high-profile case that raised issues about the fairness of the organ allocation system was that of Mickey Mantle, a retired baseball star and well-known public figure. Mantle was well known both during his career and following retirement as a drinker and a partier. However, he received treatment for alcoholism at the Betty Ford Center, a substance abuse treatment center in California, beginning in January 1994, and he had ceased consuming alcohol by the time of his release. At that time, Mantle had been told by a physician that his liver was damaged by cirrhosis due to years of high alcohol consumption, and it was later learned that he had liver cancer as well. In June 1995, he received a liver transplant at the Baylor University Medical Center in Texas and died on August 13, 1995. The apparent speed with which Mantle received his transplant, that he received it despite years of alcohol abuse (which damages the liver) and despite having liver cancer, caused many to question whether he received favorable treatment as a celebrity. Cancer patients are typically not good candidates for an organ donation, because the immunosuppressive drugs that must be taken following transplant reduce the body's ability to identify and destroy cancer cells. Mantle's short survival time following transplant (about three months) also caused some to question if giving him a donor liver was the best choice for so scarce a resource. However, the medical professionals involved in his case said that all the correct procedures were followed in allocating the liver to Mantle and that the extent of his cancer was not known at the time the transplant was performed.

The number of organs successfully transplanted increases each year, in many cases resulting in an increased life span and improved quality of life for the organ recipients. There is one limiting factor in organ transplantation, however—the availability of suitable organs to be transplanted. Despite an increase in donations, thanks in part to public education campaigns, demand for donor organs has far outstripped supply in many countries. Given that donor organs are a scarce resource, and that the question of organ transplantation involves matters of life and death, organ allocation systems have been developed to match organs with recipients as fairly as possible. What is fair is partly a question of values and ethics, and there are multiple factors to consider in devising a system of allocation that most people will accept as just and equitable. Maintaining public belief in the integrity of the organ allocation process is important because registering as a donor is an altruistic act, and people who feel the system is not just and fair may be less inclined to sign up as a donor.

CHAPTER 8

Legal Issues in Organ Donation

Organ donation and transplantation is governed by law in most countries, with strict procedures in place to ensure that donations are truly voluntary and that organs are allocated to recipients in a fair manner (both statements are open to interpretation, of course). In particular, it is illegal in almost all countries to buy and sell human organs. However, the demand for organs far exceeds the supply obtained through altruistic donations, and it is not surprising that an unofficial, extralegal "black market" has arisen to meet some of this demand. This chapter examines the black market in organs, trafficking in human organs, transplant tourism, and organ harvesting from prisoners. It should be noted that because the activities in question are generally illegal and also broadly considered unethical, information about them must often be gained from nongovernmental sources, including eye-witness testimony.

BLACK MARKETS AND TRAFFICKING IN HUMAN ORGANS

The demand for donor organs exceeds the supply, and the normal mechanisms of the marketplace usually do not apply to organ donation, because it is illegal in almost every country to buy or sell human organs. Many countries have developed systems of organ allocation that attempt to balance practical concerns with the principles of ethics and justice. In addition, there are huge differences in wealth both between and within countries. Given these conditions, it is not surprising that a black market in human organs exists in some countries or that organ trafficking is practiced in some parts of the world.

The term "black market," also referred to as a shadow or underground market, refers to economic activity (buying and selling) that exists outside the normal, government-sanctioned channels. Black markets exist for a number of reasons—for instance, because the goods being bought and sold are illegal, because the sellers wish to avoid government regulations, because the buyers and sellers wish to avoid paying taxes, or because government officials are corrupt and the market participants wish to avoid any contact with them. When a legal market is not possible, as in the case of human organs, a black market may arise to meet the demand. In some countries, particularly those with a low level of economic development and widespread poverty, the existence of black markets may be so common as to form an entire shadow economy, which may rival the official economy in terms of goods and money exchanged. In the case of donor organs, the existence of a black market is problematic for many reasons, including the lack of regulation and oversight, the bypassing of any considerations of fairness or medical necessity in favor of allocating organs based on the ability to pay, and the possibility that impoverished people may be motivated to sell their organs for cash, potentially damaging their health in the process.

While a black market is usually considered to take place in a particular area, such as a city, the term trafficking is used to refer to the movement of illegal goods over long distances, sometimes crossing national boundaries. Trafficking often serves as the supply chain for a black market. In drug trafficking, to take one example, illegal drugs are transported from their point of origin (where the drugs are grown or manufactured) to the marketplace where they are sold. So, opium grown in Afghanistan may be processed into heroin, which is then transported to the United States or Europe, where it is sold. The black market in organs, and the process of organ trafficking, is similar, including the fact that the "goods" sold (human organs) usually originate in poor countries, but are typically sold to people from rich countries.

Because organ trafficking and sale is illegal nearly everywhere, it is difficult to know how large the trade in human organs really is or exactly how it is organized. According to a 2015 report to the European Parliament, the first reports on human organ trafficking date from the 1980s and involve primarily residents of India selling their kidneys for transplantation to patients from the Gulf States, Malaysia, and Singapore. In 1994, India outlawed the buying and selling of human organs, but the trade continued. There is evidence of North American and Europeans also traveling to India to receive a donor organ, although it is difficult to determine the extent of this activity because of its illegality. After 2000, organ trafficking spread to Russia and Eastern Europe, in part due to elaborate arrangements in which a donor from an Arab country, a recipient from Israel, and a transplant surgeon from Israel, would all travel to a third country where the transplant would be carried out. There are also reports of individuals traveling from Eastern European countries to Turkey in order to donate their organs in return for payment; in some cases, the "donation" may have been coerced.

According to the 2015 report to the European Parliament, in 2007 the World Health Organization estimated that from 3,400 to 6,800 kidney transplants annually were performed with purchased donor organs, representing 5–10% of the total kidney transplants for that year. A more recent estimate of 5,000–7,000 commercial kidney transplants is also stated in the 2015 report. Organ trafficking has also become more widespread since 2000, with reports of the illegal organ trade in countries as diverse as Costa Rica, Columbia, Egypt, Lebanon, and Vietnam. One factor motivating the expansion of organ trafficking is the increased demand for organs due to the increasing number of countries where organ transplantation is now offered as a medical procedure and the correspondingly greater number of transplants performed each year. Another possible factor is the global financial crisis of 2007–2009, which acted alongside poverty and political and social unrest to increase the number of people desperate enough for money to undertake the risks of live donation.

Because of the short amount of time during which an organ is viable for transplant after removal from the donor's body, in the past typically, people seeking a transplant would travel to the country where the donor lived, and the surgery would be performed there. The recipient would then travel back to his or her home country, where they would receive aftercare. However, a different method has since become more common, in which the donor is brought to the recipient's country, or to a third location, before the organ is removed; this is called trafficking of human beings for the removal of organs (THBOR). A related topic, transplant tourism (in which an individual travels to another country in order to receive an organ transplant), will be covered in the next section.

Reasons cited in the 2015 report for seeking a kidney on the black market included long waitlists for a donated organ, lack of eligibility for a donor organ due to a health condition, replacing a failing organ before it ceases to function (e.g., someone with kidney disease seeking a transplant to avoid beginning dialysis), not wanting to ask relatives to consider a live donation, living in a country where transplantation was not available, or believing that one would be discriminated against in the organ allocation process in one's home country. Characteristics common among people selling their organs included poverty, coming from an undeveloped country, being in a position of vulnerability (e.g., an illegal immigrant), having a low education level, being unaware of the risks of donating a kidney, being male, being in age range 18–30, and coming from a country marked by government corruption. In addition, some people selling their organs reported being coerced into the transaction or being lured into it through fraud.

Organ trafficking in all its forms has been denounced by multiple international organizations. In 1985, the World Medical Association issued a *Statement on Live Organ Trade*, denouncing the sale and purchase of human organs for transplantation and calling on government to take steps to prevent organ trafficking. In 2000, the United Nations issued the *Palermo Protocol*, which defined the trafficking in human beings as a crime. In 2008, *The Declaration of Istanbul on Organ Trafficking and Transplant Tourism* was developed at a summit convened by the International Society of Nephrology and The Transplantation Society; this Declaration was updated in 2018. The European Union issued a directive in 2011 on preventing and combatting human trafficking, and in 2014, the Council of Europe issued the *Convention on Action against Trafficking in Human Beings*. However, efforts to end organ trafficking come up against the same difficulties that plague efforts to prevent many other types of crime, such as drug trafficking—the networks are international and are run by experienced criminals, large numbers of motivated buyers and sellers exist, and the illegal trade provides something that is not attainable through normal market procedures. As with other types of human trafficking, organ trafficking exploits imbalances in power—the sellers are mostly poor and disenfranchised, the buyers rich and powerful—and governments tend to favor the interests of the latter group over the former. In addition, those imbalances are unlikely to be abolished any time soon.

TRANSPLANT TOURISM

Transplant tourism is a subset of medical tourism, in which a person travels to a foreign country to receive medical care. Medical tourism is increasingly common for individuals from developed countries, and it may be motivated by the differences in cost between, for instance, having hip replacement surgery in India versus the same surgery in the United States. Another reason for medical tourism may be that an individual would want a procedure to be performed, such as plastic surgery or bariatric (weight loss) surgery, that is not covered by their insurance. World-class medical care is available today in many countries, and there is no reason to object to medical tourism *per se* as a way to receive medical care. Some American insurance companies, for instance, offer medical tourism as a choice for procedures such as hip replacement, and they cover the insured person's travel costs as well as the medical costs of the procedure, because the total cost would still be comparable or lower than having the procedure performed in an American hospital.

If the medical procedure involved is an organ transplant, the ethical issues become more difficult to resolve. This is particularly the case when the process involves the organ recipient traveling from a rich country, where organ transplant services are available and an allocation system for donor organs is in place, to a poor country where the transplant takes place. The problem with this type of medical tourism, often called transplant tourism, is that the organ to be transplanted may have been purchased, contrary to the laws of the country where the transplant takes place, or may have been obtained through coercion. In a poor country, the very fact of paying thousands of dollars for a human organ (most often a kidney) could be considered coercion, because the amount of money offered is more than the individual selling their organ could possibly earn through normal means. Another issue that arises in transplant tourism is the possibility the donor organ may have been removed from an executed prisoner without their consent. Because of the likelihood of coercion or the illegal purchase of donor organs, transplant tourism is therefore considered a type of organ trafficking (it is named as such in the Declaration of Istanbul, for instance).

One type of transplant tourism that is generally considered legitimate is when a person from a country where organ transplant services are not available (for anyone) travels to a country where such services are available to receive a transplant. For instance, a person from a country with a relatively undeveloped medical system, where organ transplants are not a possibility, might travel to a country such as the United States to receive an organ transplant. Assuming normal procedures are followed in the country where the transplant is performed, this process simply allows a person to receive a potentially lifesaving procedure that is not available in their home country. However, some question the decision to allocate a scarce donor organ to a foreign national while residents of the country where the transplant takes place must remain on transplant waiting lists, where some will die without receiving an organ.

This practice of allowing organ transplants to foreign national recipients is examined by David Goldberg and Thomas Schiano with regard to liver transplants in the United States. They note that there are no U.S. laws prohibiting performing organ transplants on foreign nationals, and even the "5% rule," which allowed for auditing of any transplant center with more than 5% of their annual transplants performed on foreign nationals, does not carry any type of enforcement. They examined medical records for adult deceased donor liver transplants (DDLT) performed in the United States from 2005 through 2013 and determined that, depending on the criteria used to define "foreign national," from 314 to 366 DDLTs were performed on foreign nationals in the United States during those years (on average, 34.9–40.7 per year). In a context of fewer than 6,000 DDLTs performed each year in the United States, and about 2,500 liver waitlist removals due to death or deteriorating health, they question whether allocating donor livers to foreign nationals is the best use of a scarce resource. They also note that, if the practice of allocating donor organs to foreign nationals were widely known, it might reduce trust in the allocation system and discourage individuals from registering to be donors. At the same time, they acknowledge that a ban on transplants to foreign nationals would deny some people lifesaving treatment, so the issue is a difficult one.

The more worrisome type of transplant tourism involves the purchase of organs for transplant, in violation of commonly held ethical principles and in most countries a violation of the law as well. As with other types of organ trafficking, it is not possible to know exactly how many people take part in transplant tourism each year. The individuals directly involved in the transplant have no reason to ask too many questions about how the organ was obtained, and those involved in obtaining the organ have no reason to make their activities known, because they are usually violating local laws. Medical professionals in the recipient's home country, where they receive aftercare, are obligated to provide medical care to their patients, and not ask questions about how an organ transplant was obtained. However, given the demand for donor organs, and the differences in wealth that exist worldwide, it is not surprising that transplant tourism exists. In fact, a 2019 article in *Infectious Disease News* offered an estimate that 10% of organ transplants each year involve an organ obtained through transplant tourism.

A few studies conducted in the United States and Canada indicate that the recipients of organs through transplant tourism are usually male and well educated and return to the country of their birth for the organ transplant. For instance, one study cited by *Infectious Disease News* looked at 93 people in British Columbia who had obtained a kidney through transplant tourism: 90% were members of ethnic minority groups (relative to the Canadian population as a whole) who returned to their country of origin for the transplant. Because that study was not based on a random sample, however, it is not possible to generalize the results to the entire Canadian population. Reasons for seeking a transplant overseas included lower costs and less waiting time.

One concern with transplant tourism is the possibility of medical complications, including infections at the surgical site (a particular worry in countries where multidrug-resistant organisms are prevalent), the risk of blood-borne fungal and viral infections, and the receipt of an organ that has not been screened for diseases such as HIV, Hepatitis B, and Hepatitis C. As the organ recipient typically returns to his home country for medical care following the transplant, these costs are imposed on the national medical system or on his or her insurance company.

The medical risks of transplant tourism were examined more closely by Daniel Fu-Chang Tsai and colleagues in a 2017 article. They compared outcomes for kidney and liver transplant recipients for Taiwanese residents, performed either in Taiwan or overseas, over an 11-year period from 1998 to 2009. This study included 2381 domestic kidney transplant recipients, 2518 overseas kidney transplant recipients, 1750 domestic liver transplant recipients, and 540 overseas liver transplant recipients; almost all of the overseas kidney and liver transplants took place in China. Overall, recipients of overseas transplants, both kidney and liver, were older and more likely to be male than recipients of domestic transplants. In addition, overseas kidney transplant recipients had a shorter pre-op dialysis period and more comorbidities in comparison to domestic kidney transplant recipients, and overseas liver transplant recipients were more likely to have hepatocellular carcinoma as compared to domestic transplant recipients.

For both kidney and liver transplants, patient survival rates were significantly greater for those receiving domestic rather than overseas transplants, with differences in survival increasing as the time from transplant increased. For kidney transplants, the 1-year survival rate (the percentage of transplant recipients alive one year after the transplant was performed) was 96.9% for domestic transplants, versus 95.8% for overseas transplants; the 5-year survival rates were 91.7% and 87.8%, respectively, and the 10-year survival rates were 83.0% and 73.1%, respectively. For liver transplants, the 1-year survival rates were 89.2% for domestic transplants and 79.8% for overseas; the 5-year survival rates were 79.5% and 54.7%, respectively, while the 10-year survival rates were 75.2% and 49.9%, respectively. The authors note that some of the differences in survival could be attributed to the overseas transplant recipients, who are on average older, being more likely to have other conditions that threatened their survival.

HARVESTING ORGANS FROM PRISONERS

Transplant tourism is dependent on the availability of donor organs for transplant. Since donor organs are a scarce resource, and demand exceeds supply, different methods have been used to try to increase the number of donor organs available for transplant. One method, which is discussed most often with reference to China, is the harvesting of organs from executed prisoners. Chinese law does not specifically outlaw the harvest of organs from condemned prisoners, and it is possible that some prisoners would voluntarily agree to donate their organs. However, medical ethics regards such "voluntary donations" as inherently problematic due to the imbalance of power between the prisoner and whoever is seeking their agreement, and there were reports from China that condemned prisoners would receive better treatment if they agreed to donate their organs. The question of coercion has also been raised with regard to medical research being performed on prisoners, for the same reason—the condition of being incarcerated places limits on how voluntary any action by the prisoner can be considered to be.

According to a 2007 report by the Transplantation Society, an international organization headquartered in Montreal, while organ transplantation was first developed and implemented as routine health care in the United States, Europe, and Australia, China has since developed one of the largest transplant programs in the world. In 2005, for instance approximately 11,000 organ transplantations were performed in China. Since the 1980s, there has been suspicion, on the part of some international organizations, that many of the organs obtained from transplant in China were obtained from prisoners who had been executed. The Chinese government has since acknowledged that this was a fact. There have also been reports from the early 1990s that organs for transplantation were being bought and sold in China and that Chinese hospitals were advertising internationally to attract foreigners seeking an organ transplant to come to China for the procedure (i.e., the hospitals were encouraging transplant tourism).

Obtaining organs from executed prisoners is condemned by the Transplantation Society, because it believes that such donations are not truly voluntary and since the 1990s has stipulated that none of its members should be involved in either obtaining or transplanting organs harvested from executed prisoners. Buying and selling human organs is also condemned by many international organizations. These ethical declarations, however, have no legal force. It is also worth noting that the buying of selling of human organs and the harvesting of organs from an executed prisoner for transplant into anyone other than a relative of the prisoner are both illegal in China. Because both practices are illegal, it would not be reasonable to expect any official records of them to exist, and it would be expected that people involved in both practices would have every incentive to conceal their behavior.

According to a 2017 report by Simon Denyer, China has acknowledged that formerly the practice of harvesting organs from prisoners who had been condemned to death was followed but that that practice has ceased. This admission confirmed what many international observers had already believed—that the rapid growth in organ transplants in China (second in volume only to the United States) was built on a system in which organs were obtained without consent and allocated based on the ability to pay rather than medical necessity. In some years, thousands of organs were harvested from prisoners and used in transplantation. This change in policy is attributed in large part to the creation of an alternative, voluntary system of organ donation over a 10-year period, primarily due to the efforts of a Chinese official, Huang Jiefu, in cooperation with an American transplant surgeon, Michael Millis.

It may never be possible to determine how many organs were harvested from condemned prisoners in the past in China, and it is also difficult to know if the practice has entirely ceased, because the Chinese government has not made that information available (and they would have nothing to gain by doing so). The other interested parties, in particular, the recipient of a donated organ and the surgeons who perform the transplant, also have no reason to ask too many questions about where the donor organ came from and whether proper legal guidelines were followed. It has therefore been left to outside organizations to investigate organ harvesting in China and to attempt to determine the extent of this practice.

In 2006, an investigation by two Canadian citizens, David Matas (a human rights lawyer) and David Kilgour (former Secretary of State for the Asia Pacific Region), reported that donor organs had been obtained involuntarily from Falung Gong practitioners and that the donors were deliberately killed during or after the surgery (so they were not executed due to being convicted of a crime, but killed for their organs). Their bodies were cremated afterward, so their corpses could not be examined or the source of the organs identified. The Transplant Society found the report of Matas and Kilgour, based on interviews conducted outside China plus analysis of written reports, to be sufficiently alarming to ask the World Health Organization to investigate the matter further.

If the allegations are true, they would represent an example of a minority group, in this case a minority following a specific spiritual practice, being victimized due to their membership in that group. According to Matas and Kilgour, Falun Gong was founded in 1992 by Li Hongzhi, as a practice that incorporated aspects of Buddhism, Confucianism, and Taoism. Falun Gong was not meant to be a political movement, but promotes truth, tolerance, and passion; members follow specific meditation, exercise, and breathing practices. However, as the popularity of Falun Gong increased (there were an estimated 70 million adherents in China in 1999), the Chinese government began to perceive it as a threat, and Falun Gong was banned in July 1999. Since then, there have been many reports of human rights abuses in China being directed toward Falun Gong practitioners, including imprisonment and torture. It is difficult to establish specifics regarding the extent of this abuse, however, as the Chinese government has no legal obligation to provide information on this matter.

THE CHINA TRIBUNAL

A more recent investigation suggests that the practice of forcibly harvesting organs from Falung Gong practitioners and members of other minority groups, including Uyghur Muslims, continues to be practiced in China. The China Tribunal is an independent judicial investigation commissioned by the International Coalition to End Transplant Abuse in China (ETAC), a not-for-profit coalition of lawyers, academics, medical professionals, and human rights advocates. The British lawyer Sir Geoffrey Nice, QC, chaired the China Tribunal, which in 2019 issued a report on forced organ donation in China and followed that with its *Final Judgment* in March 2020. The *Final Judgment* describes the China Tribunal as an investigation by citizens into an important issue not being dealt with by other national or international bodies and likens their work to that of the "Comfort Woman" Tribunal, which investigated the forced sexual slavery of Korean women at the hands of the Japanese.

The *Final Judgment* cites direct evidence (based on statements from individuals involved in the actions) dating as far back as 1978 of forced organ harvesting, meaning killing a person deliberately in order to remove their organs for transplant into another person, with multiple such incidents cited in the 1990s. The persons killed in this manner were nearly always prisoners condemned to death, although the *Final Judgment* also mentions a few known instances of single kidney removal not resulting in death. The *Final Judgment* cites indirect evidence (inferred from witness statements) of execution for the purpose of providing cadavers for dissection as early as 1940 and instances of organ harvesting from political prisoners dating back to 1978. It also reports that medical personnel, including physicians, were involved in many stages of the organ harvesting process, from the blood testing and physical examination of prisoners (used to determine if their organs are suitable for transplant and to determine a match with a recipient) to the carrying out of the surgery, but notes that the personnel in question would have been subject to retribution had they refused.

There are also reports of blood testing and medical examinations being forcibly conducted on minority groups, including Falun Gong practitioners, Uygher, Tibetans, and some House Christian groups (individual who gather for worship in private homes), suggesting that those religious and ethnic minorities were being targeted for forced organ extraction while they were living in the community.

Having a ready supply of organs for transplant allowed substantial growth in the practice of organ transplantation in Chinese hospitals. Determining how many hospitals in China were performing organ transplants at any time is difficult because of discrepancies in official government numbers as compared to other reports. This question is basically impossible to answer before 2007, because there was no system for hospitals to apply for government approval for performing transplants before that time. In 2007, over 1,000 hospitals applied for permits, but only 146 received them; however, there are reports of 566 other hospitals continuing to perform organ transplantation without government approval. A similar problem exists in trying to determine how many organ transplants took place in a given year in China, with official government statistics far lower than the numbers that could be computed using data from individual hospital websites, scientific papers, and similar sources.

Following a change in government policy in 2012, many more hospitals became transplant centers. Some of those are staffed by the military and police authorities and are required to be commercially viable. The provision of organ transplants to foreigners could be quite lucrative; for instance, there are reports of individuals needing a transplant paying as much as US $200,000 for a kidney and US $300,000 a liver. Individuals seeking a donor organ were apparently given an explanation, such as the donor dying in a traffic accident, for the availability of the organ. However, the fact that transplants could be prescheduled from abroad (versus being arranged hurriedly when an organ becomes available following an individual's natural death) would suggest to anyone with minimal knowledge of the usual organ donation process that something out of the ordinary was going on. The fact that potential recipients did not have to register on a waiting list, which is the usual experience in countries where voluntary organ donation after death is the rule, is also suspicious.

Using a variety of types of evidence, the Tribunal estimated that 60,000–90,000 organ transplants were carried out annually in China in the years from 2000 to 2014. This far exceeds the number of organs that could have been obtained from registered organ donors, which numbered 5,146 as of 2017 (larger than any number of donors registered between 2000 and 2014). This leads to the logical conclusion that Chinese hospitals must have had access, in large numbers, to a source of organs not coming from registered donors. They also conclude that the primary unreported source of the additional organs was Falun Gong practitioners, with some also coming from Uyghurs; both groups were subjected to routine abuse during the time period in question. The Tribunal also finds that China was guilty of genocide and crimes against humanity against Falun Gong practitioners and Uyghurs due to the killing and the causing of serious physical and mental harm to members of both groups. As such, they state that any individual, organization, or government that does business or otherwise interacts with China should be aware that China is, due to the actions described in the *Final Judgment* and the lack of evidence that such actions have ceased, a criminal state. These conclusions are shocking, but are based on an extensive investigation, with the evidence collected and the logic by which the judgment was reached both freely available on the internet (see the *Final Judgment* listed in "Directory of Resources").

THE CHINA ORGAN HARVEST RESEARCH CENTER

The China Tribunal is not the organization to present a report documenting apparent illegal organ trafficking in China. Another independent fact-finding report, "Documenting Genocide," on the same subject was presented in 2019 by the China Organ Harvest Research Center (COHRC), a nonprofit, nongovernmental organization based in the United States. COHRC was formed to investigate claims, beginning in 2006, that Falun Gong adherents in China were being deliberately killed so that their organs could be harvested for transplant. In 2018, COHRC issued a report of the results of its investigations, and the 2019 report summarizes those results as well as includes firsthand testimonies from numerous individuals, including relatives of organ harvesting victims and others who were detained but escaped organ harvesting. Much of the evidence in the COHRC is consonant with allegations in the *Final Judgment* of the China Tribunal.

The COHRC report noted that China prioritized the organ transplantation in national development strategies beginning in 2001, with renewed commitment to that industry in subsequent Five-Year Plans. This support included investment in research, training, and development. The sequence of events leading up to an organ transplant in China is different from that in most other countries. For instance, individuals seeking organ transplant in China can often schedule them in advance, and if a donor organ proves to be a mismatch, a second organ is sometimes quickly obtained. When waiting times are required, they are much shorter than is the norm elsewhere in the world.

Despite Chinese claims that organs for transplant were obtained primarily from death-row donations, and after 2015 from voluntary donations, the COHRC repots notes that the number of organs available in this way is much less than the number transplanted annually. For instance, China only established a voluntary organ donation system in 2010, and just over 200 donations were obtained in this way in the first two years of the system's existence. Several reasons are given for the limited extent of voluntary organ donation in China, including cultural prohibitions, a lack of public trust in the medical system, and the lack of legislation defining brain death. Insufficient government investment in voluntary organ donation may be another reason—for instance, as of 2017, only one person was responsible for overseeing voluntary organ donation and transplantation in the entire country.

The COHRC report states that Chinese government action against Falun Gong practitioners dates back to at least 1996, which intensified in 1999 when Falun Gong with creation of the "610 Office," also called the "Central Leading Group for Handling the Falun Gong Issue." In 2003, the 610 Office was given a second name, the "State Council Office for the Prevention and Handling of Cult-Related Issues." The 610 Office has broad, extralegal power to eliminate Falun Gong, and its operations are officially secret. However, documents issued by other agencies speak of matters such as the prohibition of Chinese Communist Party members practicing Falun Gong and later of the creation of camps for the "transformation" of Falun Gong practitioners (such transformation requires, among other things, relinquishing Falun Gong, surrendering related books and materials, and writing a repentance statement). The report cites numerous accounts of torture and mistreatment of Falun Gong practitioners, who constitute the largest group of prisoners of conscience in China.

The COHRC report cites numerous reports of Falung Gong practitioners, including those living in the community, being subjected to the types of medical testing that would be practiced if they were being considered organ donors. These tests include the collection of blood samples and cheek swabs, the latter a method of acquiring the cells needed for DNA testing. They also obtained testimony from physicians who were coerced into taking part in illegal organ harvesting from living prisoners. Finally, the need for hospitals to make a profit, following reforms in the Chinese health system in the 1990s, added motivation for hospitals to conduct organ transplants, which can be billed at high prices. The price charged for an organ transplant is not fixed at the national level and may vary according to the recipient's ability to pay, with reports of some foreign recipients paying the equivalent of several million dollars for a transplant.

The COHRC report estimates that the number of organ transplants conducted in China each year is probably close to 70,000 and certainly much higher than the official figures of 10,000–15,000. They also conclude that large numbers of foreign nationals receive organ transplants in China each year, despite resolutions, and sometimes laws, condemning transplant tourism. The large number of donor organs required for transplantation on that scale cannot be met by the official voluntary organ donation system, and the COHRC report concludes that the primary source of organs extracted without consent come from Falun Gong practitioners, with smaller numbers coming from other groups including Uyghur Muslims, Tibetan Buddhists, and House Christians. The COHRC report concludes that Falun Gong practitioners have been victims of genocide, as defined by the Geneva convention, and that China is guilty of crimes of humanity against them.

RESOLUTIONS AND LEGISLATION AGAINST ORGAN TRAFFICKING

In 2013, the European Parliament (the elected legislative body of the European Union) passed a resolution denouncing organ harvesting in China and calling on the Chinese government to end the practice of harvesting organs from members of minority groups. The resolution also called for member states to denounce organ transplant abuses in China, for release of Falun Gong and other prisoners of conscience, and for the Chinese government to allow an investigation of organ transplant practices in their country and to explain the apparent discrepancies in the number of organs transplanted annually, versus the number of donor organs available. In 2016, the House of Representatives of the United States, a federal legislative body, passed a resolution condemning forced organ harvesting in China. This resolution also called for an end to persecution of Falun Gong practitioners and called for the Department of State to conduct an investigation into Chinese organ harvesting and to prohibit the issuing of visas to anyone involved in coerced organ or tissue transplantation.

Some countries have gone further and passed laws intended to discourage their citizens from taking part in organ trafficking, even if the transplant of a trafficked organ takes place in another country. It must be remembered, however, that passage of a law is not the same as its enforcement. Israel passed the *Organ Transplant Act* in 2008, which prohibits insurance companies from reimbursing the costs of transplants received in countries that violate organ trafficking and trade guidelines in force in Israel. The same law also stipulates a fine and three years' imprisonment for taking part in the sale, purchase, or trafficking of an organ in any country in the world. Passage of this law had two results: an increase in organ donations and registered donors within Israel and cessation (according to the COHRC) of Israelis traveling to China to receive an organ transplant.

In 2010, Spain passed an amendment to their Criminal Code that imposed new penalties on anyone involved in organ trafficking. The punishments prescribed include 6–12 years of imprisonment for participating in illegal organ trafficking in vital organs and 3–6 years of imprisonment for trafficking in non-vital organs. Trafficking is defined in this amendment to include facilitating, advertising, or promoting the illegal procurement or transplantation of human organs. Recipients who knowingly accept transplant of an illegal organ are subject to the same penalties, although the penalties may be lowered, based on the circumstance involved. In addition, if an individual makes a profit in the process of engaging in organ trafficking, that person is subject to a fine of three to five times the profit made.

In 2015, Italy approved a bill that imposes penalties on individuals or takes part in the buying or selling of illegally tracked organs. This bill applies to any country in the world, but was particularly aimed at preventing Italian citizens from receiving organ transplants in China, following publicity regarding organ harvesting from prisoners in that country. An individual convicted of facilitating illegal organ donations faces penalties including 3–12 years imprisonment and fines of 50,000–300,000 euros. In addition, doctors found guilty of promoting or facilitating illegal organ tourism would lose their medical licenses.

Also in 2015, Taiwan passed the *Human Transplantation Act*, which bans the buying, selling, and brokerage of organs. The same law prohibits transplant tourism and the transplant of organs taken from executed prisoners, and it requires documentation of the country, hospital, and source of the transplanted organ(s) for any transplant performed abroad. Physicians taking part in illegal organ brokerage lose their licenses, and anyone involved in transplant tourism or organ brokerage is subject to imprisonment from 1 to 5 years.

Norway and Belgium have more recently passed laws criminalizing taking part in organ trafficking anywhere in the world. In 2017, Norway updated its transplant law to bring it in line with the Council of Europe Convention against Trafficking in Human Organs. The current law specifies penalties for anyone who takes part in the use, transport, or receipt of organs obtained illegally, with penalties up to 6 years depending on the extent of the crime. Belgium passed a law in 2019 that criminalizes commercial organ transaction in any country of the world, with penalties specified for anyone involved in such transactions, including physicians and patients seeking an organ transplant. Penalties include imprisonment of 5–10 years and fines of 750–75,000 euros, with increased penalties if the victim of organ harvesting dies as a result of the procedure.

Many laws govern organ donation and transplantation and international organization have also issued ethical guidelines regarding these practices. However, the demand for human organs suitable for transplant far exceeds the supply, and this problem cannot be resolved through normal market mechanisms since it is illegal in most countries to buy and sell organs. Given this context, it is not surprising that an unofficial, extralegal market in organs exists. Organ trafficking is an international concern today, but efforts to stop or control it run into the same problems as are faced when trying to end other types of illegal trade, including drug trafficking and human trafficking. Research into organ trafficking is complicated, because the practice is illegal almost everywhere, but there is substantial evidence that organ trafficking not only exists but also of how and where it is most commonly carried out.

CHAPTER 9

Financial Issues in Organ Donation and Transplantation

Organ transplantation can save lives, but, like any medical treatment, it costs money to provide it. The way that medical care, including organ transplantation, is paid for varies from one country to the next. This chapter will focus on the American system of health insurance and health care service delivery, which is extremely complex in comparison to that of countries that have a national system of health care delivery. Because of this complexity, the ability of an individual to pay for needed care can vary widely, based on the type of insurance they have. This means that a general description of how the process works must be read with the understanding that one person's situation with regard to health insurance may be vastly different from that of another. This chapter describes some basics of how health care is paid for in the United States and then considers how those variables affect the organ donation process. Finally, the issue of payment or other compensation to organ donors is discussed.

COST, CHARGES, AND PAYMENTS

There are many difficult health care systems in the world and many different ways of providing and paying for that care. The medical services required before, during, and after organ transplantation are no exception. It is therefore impossible to make global generalizations about the costs of organ transplantation, since those costs may differ so much from one country to the next. This chapter will focus on how such matters are handled in the United States. It should be noted that the American system of employment-linked health insurance, supplemented by various public and private plans, is not typical of most countries, and so generalizations from the American system to any other country should be made very carefully, if at all. In addition, because there are so many different types of insurance within the American system of health care, generalizing even from one person to another can be treacherous. This means that any attempt to predict the costs involved in organ transplantation for a specific individual must be determined based on the particular situation of that individual; the information provided in this chapter speaks more to financial issues in more general terms.

It should be noted that this discussion applies to those who receive donated organs, not those who donate them. Any expenses involved in the organ donation process are paid for by the individual receiving the organ, usually through their insurance company.

One distinction that is particularly relevant in the American health care context is the distinction among charges, costs, and payments. The average patient may be quite surprised to learn that there is a distinction among these terms, and they are often confused or misused in news media stories about health care. However, understanding what these terms mean to professionals in working in health care administration or in the insurance business is vital to understanding how health care, including organ transplantation, is provided and paid for in the United States. Charges refer to the price a hospital sets for providing a particular item or service, be it a simple medicine like aspirin or a complex test such as a CT scan or the provision of surgical services. These charges are stored on an internal list called a chargemaster, and charges for the identical item or service may vary widely from one hospital to another.

Charges bear no relation to the amount a hospital bills for patients covered by Medicare or Medicaid (the former a federal insurance program primarily for individuals age 65 and older, the latter a joint federal-state insurance program primarily for the poor), because the amount that can be billed in those insurance systems is standard and set at the federal level. Charges may act as a point of departure for negotiations with private insurers, however, including those providing coverage through the insured person's employer. The amount that a hospital receives can vary widely from one insurer to another, but is generally far lower than the official charge.

Uninsured patients who pay out of pocket might be billed the official charge for a procedure, but more likely will be offered a discounted price since charges are typically higher than the amount an insurer would pay for an item or service. Charges may also be relevant to individuals who receive care outside the network of hospitals and physicians included in their insurance plan, because in that situation they don't have the benefit of the lower price negotiated by their insurance company. Charges are also relevant to insured individuals because a person admitted to a hospital within their insurer's network may receive care from a physician working in the hospital but who is not included in the insurer's network; this situation can result in people receiving large "surprise bills" for services patients thought were covered by their insurance policy.

The meaning of the term "costs" is more intuitive—it refers to the actual expense a hospital incurs while providing medical care. Costs include both obvious direct costs for services and items used in patient care, such as medicines, supplies, nursing care, and food, and indirect costs that an individual patient might not be aware of, such as building maintenance, reporting to regulatory agencies, infection control procedures, and the costs of maintaining medical records. Costs may vary widely from one hospital to the next, depending on factors such as location and function of the hospital (a rural hospital that provides only a limited range of services is likely to have lower costs than an urban teaching hospital, for instance).

While some health care administrators regard the chargemaster system as an irrelevant relic of a past era, a 2016 research article by Ge Bai and Gerard F. Anderson reports that the charge structure of a hospital does seem to have some relation to its costs. They looked at the charge-to-cost ratio at a number of hospitals, the charge-to-cost ratio being a measure of price markup found by dividing the chargemaster price for a given service or item for each hospital by the Medicare allowable reimbursement (which is standard across the country). They found that hospitals appeared to systematically adjust their charge-to-cost ratios, which ranged from 1.8 to 28.5 depending on the hospital department involved, with charge-to-cost ratios higher at for-profit hospitals than at nonprofit or government hospitals.

For all hospitals taken together, the charge-to-cost ratio was 4.32, with the lowest ratio of 3.47 found for government hospitals, followed by 3.79 for nonprofit hospitals, and 6.31 for for-profit hospitals. The charge-to-cost ratio was on average higher for hospitals with a high proportion of uninsured patients, system affiliated, as opposed to independent hospitals and hospitals with regional power. The highest charge-to-cost ratios were found for CT scans (28.5), anesthesiology (23.5), and MRI services (13.6), while the lowest ratios were found for general routine care (1.8), intensive care (2.1), and nursery (2.7). They suggest that costs are generally higher in departments supplying more complex services, which make it more difficult for patients and insurers to compare charges across hospitals. Higher charge-to-cost ratios were also associated with higher patient care revenue, suggesting the chargemaster prices were adjusted to maximize revenue.

A medical consumer is unlikely to be directly concerned with either hospital costs or charges, but they should know that both may influence which hospitals are included within their care network, because insurers have an incentive to limit their networks to lower-cost institutions and providers. As noted, there can be a wide variation within a single hospital in the ratio between charges and costs, with the most complex services generally having higher charge-to-cost ratios.

In the United States, insurers typically establish a network of hospitals, labs, and health care providers with whom they have negotiated rates. If an insured individual seeks care within the established network of his or her insurer, they will pay much less (sometimes nothing), while if they receive care outside that network, they may be liable for the entire cost or a much higher percentage of the cost. Insurers have an incentive to negotiate the lower possible reimbursement rates, and hospitals with high costs may demand higher reimbursement in turn for providing care. For this reason, certain hospitals or providers may not be included within the network of a particular insurance plan and therefore may effectively not be available to someone covered under that plan. The primary reason is financial: a patient's bill for hospital care not covered by their health insurance may easily run into the tens of thousands of dollars, an amount of money most people simply can't afford to pay.

The meaning of "payment" is fairly intuitive, as it refers to the money a hospital receives for providing patient care. In the United States, there are three primary sources of payments to hospitals: federal and state governments (through the Medicare and Medicaid systems), private insurance companies, and private individuals. Payments by a private individual are also referred to as "out-of-pocket payments." In addition, many insurance policies include a cost-sharing system that requires the individual receiving care to pay something for the care they receive. This may be either a fixed fee, called a copayment (e.g., a $25 copayment to see a primary care physician), or a percentage of the bill (e.g., 20% of the amount billed by the hospital for surgical services), called coinsurance. Individual insurance policies may also include a deductible so that the policy holder must pay a certain amount for care each year before the insurance policy begins paying.

FINANCIAL CONSIDERATIONS FOR THE ORGAN RECIPIENT

Because financial issues cannot be avoided when someone is seeking to become an organ transplant recipient in the United States, the United Network for Organ Sharing (UNOS) has created a guide to covering transplant costs. It begins with the caveat that every individual case is different and that anyone seeking a transplant should consult with the financial team of the transplant center where they are registered. It's also worth noting that insurance coverage can change from one year to the next (for instance, a given drug may be covered one year and not the next, and hospitals and providers may be added or dropped from the insurance company's network each year), so it is necessary to keep up with changes in one's own policy. Individuals preparing to undergo a transplant should also investigate whether they are eligible for assistance due to disability from the Social Security Administration (SSA), as discussed later, both before and after the transplant.

People outside the United States may be astonished at the complexity of the American health care system, as well as the possibility that a person's ability to access lifesaving care may be dependent on their ability to pay. On the other hand, someone always has to pay the bills, and transplant centers have to collect fees for the services they provide in order to remain in operation. The phrase "wallet biopsy" was coined to describe the financial evaluation a prospective organ recipient undergoes when attempting to register at a transplant center. In one highly publicized case, a 60-year-old woman, Hedda Martin, said she was initially turned down as a candidate for a heart transplant because she did not have sufficient financial resources or insurance coverage to buy the antirejection drugs she would need following transplant surgery. Martin raised more than $30,000 through a GoFundMe account, an online fundraising system where people can donate to various causes, and was then added to the transplant waiting list.

Many Americans, particularly those under the age of 65, have private health insurance, often through a group policy available through their employer. Many insurance companies offer coverage for transplant costs, but as with other types of medical treatment, a given insurance plan may not pay for everything, and the individual may end up paying quite a bit out of pocket. As a general rule, in the United States an individual patient is obligated to personally pay any bills presented for their care that are not covered by insurance (the patient usually signs a document accepting this responsibility before any care will be provided). Among the questions that a transplant recipient should consider are whether the transplant center is in his/her insurer's network; if not, what out of network benefits, if any, may apply; what might they have to pay in deductibles, copays, or coinsurance; if prior authorization from the insurance company is required and, if so, how to get it; if there is a lifetime maximum dollar amount that the insurance company will pay; and are there any specific rules regarding preexisting conditions.

Medicare, a federal program that provides health insurance to people age 65 or older, the disabled, and people with end-stage renal disease, will pay for transplantation services for the kidneys, the kidneys and pancreas, and under certain circumstances the pancreas alone. If the recipient is covered by Medicare due to age or disability, more types of organ transplant are covered, including the lungs, the heart (in certain circumstances), the heart and lungs, the liver, and the intestines. The transplant must take place in a Medicare-approved transplant program, and Medicare may not cover all the expenses involved with a transplant, so the recipient should determine what they will be required to pay for. Many Medicare recipients also have supplemental insurance to cover what Medicare does not, but the insured person still needs to determine if there will be additional expenses not covered by either type of insurance that they will be obligated to pay out of pocket. Coverage for prescription drugs is included in Medicare Part D, which is optional but selected by most people; this adds another layer of complexity since the individual then needs to determine if the drugs they will need before and after the transplant are covered.

Medicaid, a federal-state health insurance program, is administered differently by each state. In general, Medicaid exists to serve low-income individuals, but each state has different rules for eligibility and offers different benefits. Many Medicaid programs will cover organ transplants, but only if they are conducted within the state, with a possible exception that the state does not include a center that can transplant the organ in question. The TRICARE system, which funds medical care to the families of individuals serving or having served in the military (including retired and deceased military personnel), provides some coverage for organ transplantation, from both living and deceased donors, but the recipient must receive pre-authorization for the transplant from the TRICARE system.

Individuals who have none of the insurance coverage described above, or who will face expenses larger than they can manage even with insurance, have several other options. One is to appeal to charitable organizations, which may be able to help with some of the costs of the transplant (including ancillary expenses such as transportation and housing). Advocacy organizations may also be able to help with the costs of a transplant. A final option is to conduct a public fundraising campaign, through direct appeals to individuals and businesses, the internet (e.g., using gofundme. com or a similar website), publicity through local media, and so on. Anyone choosing this route should be careful to find out what laws and regulations apply to this type of fundraising and that the funds be used for the purpose(s) for which they were raised.

The SSA provides financial assistance to people who are unable to work due to a disability. Information about eligibility is available through the SSA website, and application for assistance can also be made through that website. Most people who have received an organ transplant are eligible for assistance for at least 12 months following surgery, and some may be eligible for longer periods. For instance, lung transplant recipients are eligible for three years of assistance following surgery. Individuals with organ failure, including those on a wait list for an organ transplant, may also be eligible for assistance; qualifying conditions include cystic fibrosis, heart failure, leukemia, liver disease, lung cancer, chronic obstructive pulmonary disease, kidney disease, and lymphoma.

ESTIMATED TRANSPLANT CHARGES AND COSTS NATIONWIDE

Milliman, an actuarial and consulting firm headquartered in Seattle, produces a number of reports concerning health care, insurance, pensions, and the like. Their 2020 report on organ and tissue transplants, authored by T. Scott Bentley and Nick J. Ortner, includes a wealth of data related to the number of transplants performed in the United States in 2020 and the average billed charges for different types of transplant, including billed charges for the period from 30 days before the transplant to 180 days after it. The estimates are based on information from the Organ Procurement and Transplantation Network, the Scientific Registry of Transplant Recipients, the Health Resources and Services Administration, and the Eye Bank of America.

Not surprisingly, multiple organ transplants carry some of the highest charges, with the single most expensive type of transplant being that of both the heart and a kidney, billed on average at $2,644,600. Heart-lung transplants were billed at the second highest amount, $2,637,200, followed by other multi-organ transplants ($2,185,800), intestine with other organs ($1,662,900), liver and kidney ($1,355,100), and kidney and pancreas ($713,800).

Among single organ transplants, a heart transplant carries the highest average billed costs at $1,664,800. Also billed at over one million dollars, on average, are a double lung transplant ($1,295,900), an intestine transplant ($1,240,700), and an allogeneic bone marrow transplant ($1,071,700; in this type of transplant, the blood stem cells transplanted come from someone other than the recipient). Average charges for other types of transplant include $929,600 for a single lung transplant, $471,600 for an autologous bone marrow transplant (in which the blood stem cells come from the individual receiving the transplant), $442,500 for a kidney transplant, $408,800 for a pancreas transplant, and $32,500 for a cornea transplant.

Detailed breakdowns of the costs for each type of transplant are available in the Milliman report (listed in "Directory of Resources"). We will look at the costs of a single type of transplant here as illustration, using the most common type of transplant, a kidney transplant, as our example. The average charges for a kidney transplant came to $442,500. Of those, $32,700 were incurred in the 30 days before transplant, including physical exams, lab tests, blood and tissue typing, cross-matching for donor compatibility, and psychological testing. Charges for procurement of the kidney average $113,900, including retrieval, preservation, and transportation of the organ. Hospital transplant admission charges averaged $152,300, including room and board, nursing care, drugs, supplies, and pathology and radiology procedures. Physician services during transplant admission averaged $26,200, including surgical procedures. Charges in the 180 days following discharge came to $140,200, including lab testing, treatment of complications, outpatient visits, and readmission if relevant. Finally, prescription charges in the 180 days following discharge averaged $31,900, including both immunosuppressant drugs and any other type of drug required in that period (antibiotics, pain medications, antianxiety drugs, etc.).

The Milliman report also breaks down the charges for different types of organ transplants in terms of PMPM or per member per month costs; that is, what each member in a plan is paying to cover the charges the insurance company pays for each type of insurance transplant. The PMPM costs are a factor of both the cost of each type of transplant and how commonly each is performed. Multiple organ transplants are among the most expensive, for instance, but are also quite rare, so the PMPM is relatively low. On the other hand, more common treatments may result in a higher PMPM charge despite a lower average cost, simply because they are more common. For instance, the highest PMPM costs are for kidney transplant, liver transplants, and allogeneic bone marrow transplants, because they are relatively common.

PAYMENT FOR ORGAN DONATION: IRAN

In most countries of the world, it is illegal to buy and sell human organs. The primary exception is Iran, which in 1988 legalized donation of kidneys to people other than relatives, with compensation provided to donors through a government-run system. At the same time, the government made substantial investments in training of medical personnel to perform transplants and in equipping and staffing hospitals so they could become transplant centers. All expenses of the transplantation process for both donor and recipient are paid for by the government, and immunosuppressant drugs are provided to the recipient following transplant at a subsidized price. Donors receive a cash payment and health insurance from the government; many also receive an additional amount of money, either from the recipient's family or from a charitable organization.

To oversee the process of bringing together donors and recipients, the Iranian government created an independent agency, the Dialysis and Transplant Patients Association (DTPA). The DPTA, which is separate from any government agency, is staffed by volunteers who are themselves end-stage renal patients. Individuals who need a donor kidney, and do not have a suitable donor within their family, are referred by their physician to the DPTA to begin the process of being matched with a donor. Potential donors are screened by a panel including transplant surgeons, nephrologists, and nurses, in order to determine if they are freely consenting to be a living donor (i.e., that they are not being pressured or coerced). In order to prevent transplant tourism and ensure that Iranian donor organs are used to help other Iranians, people from outside Iran are generally not permitted to receive a donor organ from an unrelated recipient. There is one exception to this rule: a foreign individual can obtain permission from the Ministry of Health to receive a transplant from an individual of their own nationality (allowing them to use the organ transplant infrastructure of Iran, which might not exist in their home country). In an effort to prevent bribes or illegal payments beyond what is provided by the government, potential donors are not legally allowed to contact anyone in the waiting list for a kidney, and no one, including medical professionals and anyone who might think of offering their services as a broker between donors and recipients, is allowed to receive special payment for arranging or carrying out a donation.

Iran created this system of kidney transplantation and payment in response to the large unmet need for donor kidneys, which resulted in so many people needing dialysis treatment that it was straining the country's resources. In the 1980s, Iran began paying for its citizens to receive transplants from living donors abroad, with most patients traveling to the United Kingdom for the process; in five years, over 400 Iranians received living transplants in this way. However, this proved to be an expensive way to provide kidney transplants, and Iran began to create its own network of renal transplantation teams, with about 100 kidney transplants performed annually in Iran from 1985 to 1987. However, the number of transplants performed in this way was insufficient in a country where over 25,000 people suffered from end-stage renal disease; in addition, many of the individuals needing dialysis lived in rural areas with limited access to medical care.

The system of paid donation proved immediately successful in terms of increasing the number of kidney transplants, which nearly doubled in the first year. It was also notably successful in terms of encouraging living kidney donation to unrelated individuals: this type of donation constituted almost 80% of the total in the first year. Iran does not have a national transplant registry, nor does it provide detailed information about transplant outcomes on a national basis, but examination of the records of one major hospital, the Hashemi Nejad Hospital (HRH) in Iran, found that about 2000 kidney transplants were performed in that hospital between 1986 and 2006. Of those transplants, about 75% involved living donors. Outcomes, in terms of both graft and patient survival, were comparable to those of other countries. During this time period, most living unrelated kidney donors were male (91%), as were most recipients of a kidney (63%), including transplants from both living and deceased donors. The age range of donors was from 21 to 37 years.

According to the Iranian government, the waiting list for kidney transplants was eliminated in 1999, and, as of 2006, more than half of the Iranians formerly suffering from end-stage renal disease had received a donor kidney that was functioning successfully. The prevalence of end-stage renal disease in 2004 remained higher in Iran than in the Middle East as a whole (370 patients per million population in Iran, 190 per million in the Middle East), but much lower than in some other countries and regions, such as Japan (2,045 patients per million), North America (1,505 patients per million), and Europe (585 per million).

Iran had no system of organ transplants from deceased donors when the paid living donor system was established. However, in April 2000, legislation was passed that allowed deceased organ donation and established brain death as a legitimate definition of death. The number of renal transplants using kidneys from deceased donors increased slowly but steadily following passage of this legislation. Kidneys from deceased donors were used in 1.8% of all kidney transplants in 2000, but had risen to 12% by 2005.

OTHER INCENTIVES FOR ORGAN DONATION

A few countries have created systems of incentives for organ donation, although they do not allow direct payment for donation. In Israel, for instance, individuals who register as organ donors receive priority should they need a donor organ themselves, as do their immediate relatives. Other countries provide enhanced financial benefits to living donors, but do not describe them as payments for the organ; usually they are framed as compensating the donor for loss of income and other expenses incurred as a result of donation.

According to a survey by Manisha Sickand and colleagues, nonmedical expenses such as travel, accommodation, dependent care, and lost wages are sometimes seen as a barrier to becoming a living organ donor. They identified 72 countries in which at least 10 living organ donations were performed on average between 2004 and 2007 and then analyzed the policies of the 40 countries for whom such information was available. In some of these 40 countries, the availability of reimbursement varied within the country (e.g., depending on the province or state). Of the 40 countries studied, 21 had reimbursement programs for living organ donors, with such programs most common in European countries and in North America and less common in South America and Asia.

Of the 21 countries with reimbursement programs, 10 had comprehensive reimbursement plans offering at least some reimbursement for travel, accommodation, meals, lost income, and child care. More countries had programs that allowed for reimbursement of some of those categories of expenses, including 19 with programs to reimburse travel expenses, 17 with programs to reimburse at least some lost income, 17 with programs to reimburse accommodation, 14 with programs to reimburse meals, and 12 with programs to reimburse child care costs. In 10 of the countries, reimbursement was available to people outside the province, state, or country.

In the United States, living organ donors have been eligible since 1984 to receive reimbursement for the costs of travel, lodging, meals, and incidental expenses related to organ donation. The categories of expenses eligible for reimbursement were expanded in September 2020 through the Executive Order on Advancing American Kidney Health to include lost wages, child care costs, and costs for elder care. The purpose of this new expansion of reimbursement categories was to remove financial barriers to becoming a living donor, and thus to encourage more people to become living kidney donors and to reduce the number of people on waiting lists for kidney transplants.

In Australia, the Supporting Living Organ Donors Program provides financial support to Australian residents who want to donate a kidney or partial liver within Australia. The goals of the program are to remove cost as a barrier to living organ donation, raise the profile of living organ donors, and encourage employer support of living organ donors. Australia has a universal public health insurance program, Medicare, providing free care in public hospitals and reduced cost services for other types of care. However, becoming a living organ donor requires major surgery, with the corresponding risks and potentially long recovery time. A living donor will probably need to take time off work to recover and may lose some of their salary as a result. In addition, they may have to pay for some of the expenses of donation out of pocket.

To prevent these two factors from being a barrier to donation, the program provides living donors with up to 342 hours of paid leave at the national minimum wage and reimbursement for any out-of-pocket medical expenses incurred as a result of donation. The program also provides payments to the employer of the donor, to recredit any sick leave the donor may have taken for reasons related to donation, and to reimburse the employer if the employer paid them without charging the time against their annual leave or sick leave. Individuals who are not working, including retirees, can claim up to $1,000 for expenses related to living organ donation, while those who incurred expenses or lost time from work but did not become a donor can seek reimbursement for incurred costs plus up to 72 hours of leave taken during the process preparatory to donation.

Singapore uses a similar system to encourage living organ donations and reimburse the donor for any costs, including lost wages, incurred as a result of the donation. The Human Organ Transplant Act (HOTA), enacted in 1987, legalized kidney and partial liver transplants from living donors for the first time. The process should take place in a hospital and requires written authorization by the hospital's transplant ethics team and the full and informed consent of the donor. Buying and selling of organs is prohibited by HOTA, but the law allows living donors to be compensated for medical expenses related to the donation and for lost wages during the donation and recovery period.

It would be nice if we could deal with issues of medical care, including organ transplantation, without considering the costs and who will pay them, but that's not possible in our current world. This chapter focuses on the United States with regard to the expenses of hospital care and organ transplantation, with some information about other countries as well. The American system of health care financing and delivery is extraordinarily complex, and insurance coverage can vary widely from one person to the next. For this reason, we should have the directly relevant information when making decisions about financial matters related to health care. Different countries, and sometimes different regions within the same country, have reached different conclusions on ethical issues related to the finances of organ transplantation, including whether organs can be directly bought and sold and whether compensation for expenses is available to living organ donors.

CHAPTER 10

Ethical Issues in Organ Donation

There are many ethical issues regarding organ transplantation. Many of them have their roots in scarcity, beginning with the fact there are not enough donor organs to meet the current demand for them. In addition, since the United States does not have a system of universal health care, some individuals may not be eligible to get on the waiting list for a transplant, if they do not have sufficient insurance to pay for the procedure. The allocation system is not perfect, and some have questioned whether physicians may be gaming the system to move their patients up the waiting list. Due to the shortage of donor organs, the strict standards normally applied concerning organs suitable for transplant may be relaxed, but recipients are always informed and must consent to receiving a less than ideal organ. Donors, recipients, and the families of recipients are all entitled to their privacy, and if any party wishes to contact the other, this should be arranged through an Organ Procurement Organization in order to protect confidentiality. Xenotransplantation, in which cells, tissues, or organs are transplanted across species, offers a potentially inexhaustible supply of donor organs for humans, but it also raises ethical concerns and poses the possibility of engendering the creation of infectious "super bugs."

DECEASED DONORS AND THE SUPPLY OF ORGANS FOR TRANSPLANT

The organ transplantation process requires that a suitable donor organ be available. Some may find it surprising that donor organs are in such short supply, given the millions of people who have signed up to be organ donors. Programs intended to encourage people to sign up as organ donors seldom mention the fact that most registered donors will not actually become organ donors (although they may be able to donate tissues), because the manner in which they die makes their organs unusable for transplantation. In fact, according to the Health Resources and Services Administration, about 3 in 1000 people in the United States die in a way that allows their organs to be transplanted.

Most deceased organ donors are declared dead due to brain death, meaning that they would have completely lost all brain function in a way that is irreversible, although assistance by machines and/or medications may keep their heart beating and thus the blood flowing to their organs, while a mechanical ventilator can keep them supplied with oxygen. This means that the person's organs continue to be supplied with oxygen and nutrients, as if the person were still alive, and thus the organs do not deteriorate as they rapidly do as soon as a person's heart stops beating. Brain death is relatively rare, occurring in less than 1% of all cases of death in the United States, and most cases of brain death occur in one of a few ways, including brain injury due to trauma (e.g., a head injury suffered in a traffic accident), stroke (when the blood supply to the brain is diminished due to a burst blood vessel or blockage by a blood clot), or asphyxiation (e.g., suicide by hanging).

Normally, when death is due to the cessation of heart functions (cardiac death), the organs deteriorate quickly and are thus not suitable for transplant. A patient who suffers cardiac death may be able to donate body tissues, however. In addition, it is sometimes possible for organs to be donated by someone who has suffered cardiac death, although organs donated in this way may have suffered some amount of oxygen deprivation. However, given the rarity of brain death and the shortage of donor organs, donation after cardiac death (DCD) is seen as a possible way to increase the number of organs available for transplantation. A potential DCD donor is someone who is near death from a severe and irreversible brain injury, but does not meet the formal criteria for brain death. In the case of DCD, the patient's family must consent to have care withdrawn, and the patient's organs are removed after their heart has stopped beating. To avoid even the slightest appearance of conflict of interest, the surgeons who remove the organs for transplant cannot be part of the patient's care team or be involved in the declaration of death.

DCD is divided into two categories, depending on several factors including the age of the donor and the cause of his or her death. Standard criteria donors (SCD) are under age 50, while expanded criteria donors (ECD) are over the age of 60, or are over the age of 50 and have two health conditions that might complicate the viability of their organs; these conditions include high blood pressure, death from a stroke, or a creatinine test result greater than 1.5. A recipient must consent in writing to receive a transplant from an ECD, in part because such transplants have a somewhat lower success rate than a transplant from a SCD.

In the case of kidney transplants, sometimes both kidneys from a patient with limited kidney function can be transplanted into a single patient (a dual kidney transplant); together, the two kidneys may function as effectively as a single kidney donated from someone with normal kidney function. In addition, although a child's kidney may not be sufficient to support the needs of an adult, the transplant of both kidneys from a pediatric donor into an adult (pediatric *en bloc* transplant) has been performed successfully. However, because children have smaller blood vessels than adults, kidney transplants from a child to an adult carry a slightly higher risk of vascular complications.

CERTIFICATION OF BRAIN DEATH

Brain death has been recognized in the United States since 1981, when the president's Commission for the Study of Ethical Issues in Medicine developed a definition of it. People who do not work in medicine sometimes fear that the determination of "brain death" is subjective, but in fact, it is clinically defined. A person who is brain dead has no electrical activity in their brain, as determined by an electroencephalograph (EEG). They also have a complete absence of blood flow to the brain, as determined by the injection of radioactive isotopes. This differentiates brain death from the condition of being in a coma or persistent vegetative state, because people in the latter two conditions still have electrical activity in their brain. A person who is brain dead will not have lung function, except as assisted by a respirator, and has no response to pain or light and has no gag reflex.

People sometimes fear that if they are registered as an organ donor, this may affect the type or quality of care they will receive. This is not the case: an individual who is registered as an organ donor receives exactly the same care as one who is not registered as a donor. Every possible effort is made to save the person's life, as would be the case for any patient, and care is never withdrawn to hasten a donor's death or to see that they die in a manner so that their organs can be donated. While the patient is living, therefore, their status as a potential organ donor has no influence on their medical treatment. As a further safeguard, many hospitals require two physicians to independently run a series of tests and determine that brain death has occurred. Neither physician can be involved in the organ transplant process and may not even know that the patient is a potential organ donor.

As noted earlier, brain death is a relatively recent concept, and some people find it confusing. It is important to realize that a person who is brain dead is actually dead, and there is no way that they could be brought back to life. A person's heart may stop beating and then be "shocked" back to functioning by a defibrillator, but there is no such treatment to cause a brain to resume functioning. A person who is brain dead may appear to be alive, due to mechanical support that can keep their blood circulating and supply them with oxygen, but they are in fact dead, and removing the mechanical supports therefore cannot cause their death.

MEDICAL CONTRAINDICATIONS TO ORGAN DONATION

One concern in organ transplantation is that a donor organ should not be infected by a disease that could be transmitted to the recipient. For this reason, both donor screening and lab testing are used to determine if a donor's organs are suitable for transplant. In the United States, the Organ Procurement and Transplantation Network (OPTN) is responsible for policies regarding screening of organ donors, while the Food and Drug Agency (FDA) issues regulations for tissue and eye banks. In both cases, the process of approving a donor includes conducting a medical and social history interview with the next of kin or another individual who is knowledgeable regarding the deceased. The donor's medical history will also be examined to see if they had any disease or other medical condition that would contraindicate donating their organs, and their recent travel history will also be consulted to determine if the donor might have been exposed to certain pathogens that are not prevalent in their home community.

Extensive laboratory testing is also conducted before organ donation. Current OPTN policy requires testing for HIV, hepatitis B, hepatitis, syphilis, cytomegalovirus (CMV), and Epstein Barr virus for both living and deceased donors. Deceased donors are also tested for toxoplasmosis, and living kidney donors are tested for tuberculosis if they are judged at increased risk for that disease. Tissue and eye banks are required to test donor specimens for HIV, hepatitis B, hepatitis C, and syphilis. Living donors are also tested for West Nile Virus, and donors of tissues containing live white blood cells (e.g., umbilical cord blood, semen) are also tested for CMV and human T-lymphotropic virus (HTLV).

Due to the shortage of donor organs, sometimes organs are allowed to be transplanted despite not meeting the usual medical requirements:

these are referred to as expanded criteria organs. For instance, in 2013, the United States passed the *HIV Organ Policy Equity Act* (HOPE Act), which allowed HIV-positive recipients to receive organs from HIV-positive donors. Specific protocols must be followed for this type of transplant, including a study team comprising an experienced transplant physician and physician experienced in the treatment of HIV. A similar line of reasoning means that organs from donors who are positive for hepatitis B and/or hepatitis C can be transplanted into people having those conditions, and in some cases, the transplant may be allowed even if the recipient does not have the infection in question. Other types of expanded criteria include accepting organs from donors older than usual and accepting organs from donors who have medical conditions such as hypertension that would ordinarily be disqualifying.

The use of expanded criteria organs raises its own set of ethical issues. The primary reason for allowing transplantation of expanded criteria organs is to increase the number of organs available for transplant and therefore the number of people whose lives may be saved through replacement of a failing organ. However, it would be unethical to deliberately harm the recipient by giving them a substandard organ, as that would be wasting resources on transplant operations without expectation of good outcomes for the recipient. However, for some people, receiving a functioning if compromised organ may be preferable to their current condition. In any case, the potential recipient must give informed consent to receive an expanded criteria kidney, after being informed of the risks and benefits as indicated by the most recent available research. The use of expanded criteria organs should also be conducted in a way that minimizes risk, for instance by matching organs from a donor with a particular infection to a recipient with the same infection.

Some studies have indicated that receiving an expanded criteria organ produces benefits similar to those of receiving a standard criteria organ, while others indicate that those receiving expanded criteria organs have more postoperative complications and that the organs function less effectively than standard criteria organs. The use of expanded criteria organs has been studied primarily with kidneys, which constitute the most common type of organ transplant. Because dialysis can be used to keep a patient alive while they are waiting for a donation, a choice must be made whether to compare outcomes for receiving an expanded criteria kidney against continuing with dialysis while on the waiting list, with the ultimate chance to receive a standard criteria kidney. The benefits of receiving a quicker transplant with an expanded criteria kidney must thus be weighed against the harm of losing the opportunity to receive a standard criteria kidney after a longer wait.

As summarized by James Childress and colleagues, receiving an expanded criteria kidney, as compared to remaining on dialysis, generally improves outcomes, particularly for some categories of patients. They found that mortality was 17% lower for individuals receiving an expanded criteria kidney, as compared to remaining on dialysis, with higher benefit for those older than 40 or those who had diabetes or hypertension. They suggest that expanded criteria kidneys be offered to those older than 40 and who face long waiting times for a standard criteria kidney. They also recommend that recipients facing shorter waiting times are better served by remaining on the waiting list for a standard criteria kidney. The key exception to these rules is that individuals suffering from diabetes as well as kidney failure are better served by receiving an earlier transplant of an expanded criteria kidney, rather than waiting for a standard criteria kidney.

IS THE ORGAN ALLOCATION PROCESS FAIR?

There are not enough donor organs to supply one to every person needing a transplant; most people requiring an organ are placed on a waiting list. An allocation system is used to describe who gets priority on the waiting list and ultimately who gets an organ. Given the shortage of donor organs, there is no way to create an organ allocation system that will make everyone happy, but we can ask whether the system in place in the United States is fair. Of course, what is "fair" depends in part on the values of the person making the judgment, and one's place in the process may also influence judgment—people who get an organ quickly are likely to be happy with the current system, while those who have to wait for years, who die without receiving a transplant, or who are excluded from the allocation process entirely may well have more criticisms of how the current system works.

The first issue in organ allocation is simple: who should be placed on the waiting list? If an individual is not allowed on a waiting list, they will not receive an allocated organ and are thus extremely unlikely to receive a transplant within the United States. While rules are necessary, and there may be good reasons for each rule, they can also act to discriminate against some people. For instance, most transplant centers in the United States will not accept a patient without health insurance. While there is a practical reason for this choice (medical care is expensive to provide, and the United States does not have a national health system), it might be considered unethical because it discriminates against the poor and disenfranchised. In addition, this rule has a disproportionate impact on some groups of individuals, such as African Americans, who are more likely than white Americans to be uninsured.

Age can also be a disqualifying factor, and age 75 is often used as a cutoff for being placed on a waiting list. There are good medical arguments for this rule—older people tend to be in poorer health and to have fewer expected years of life remaining, and prioritizing younger people may result in greater benefit, in terms of years of healthy life gain, for each organ transplanted. On the other hand, many people over the age of 75 are in good health and could be expected to undergo the transplant with no difficulties and to live for perhaps decades following transplant surgery, so automatically excluding people on the basis of age could be seen as an unethical form of discrimination.

Certain medical conditions or life histories may also cause a person to be excluded from the transplant waiting lists. For instance, a history of addiction, mental health difficulties, mental retardation, and an extensive criminal record have all been cited as reasons a person might be excluded. In the case of mental retardation or a history of mental health issues, the concern is that the individual might not be able to cope with the transplant process or follow the necessary medical regime following transplant. However, with appropriate support (not a given in the United States, due to our lack of a national health care system), such individuals might be able to cope as well as someone without those difficulties. And these criteria can be discriminatory, since people with sufficient wealth and/or family resources may receive the necessary support, while those who are more impoverished or lack social supports may not.

While those with active drug or alcohol additions are generally excluded from transplant consideration, due to the potential damage of those practices on the individual's health, the question of allowing recovering addicts to be included on waiting lists is more controversial. Some transplant centers will accept recovering addicts, while some will not. In some cases, individuals currently using marijuana are not accepted, even if it is legal in the state in question. Of primary concern is the possibility of the recipient relapsing into addictive behavior after receiving a transplant, thus damaging the organ and potentially needing a second transplant. It is reasonable to want to be prudent in the allocation of a scarce resource such as donor organs, but it must also be considered that addiction is more common among people who are otherwise disadvantaged in American society and that people with fewer resources are less likely to be able to receive effective treatment to fight their addiction. Looked at in this light, a reasonable decision from a medical point of view can result in yet another instance of discrimination against individuals who have already suffered much in that regard.

Exclusion on the basis of having served time in prison is generally justified not in punitive terms, but on the basis of prudent allocation of available organs. Individuals who have served time in prison may well have been exposed to more infectious diseases than those who have not and may be more likely to suffer from mental disorders or substance abuse. However, the official position of United Network for Organ Sharing (UNOS) is that convicted criminals should be considered on an individual basis, with evaluation of health and mental status being conducted as is done for any transplant candidate; status as a former prisoner should not be an automatic disqualifier. However, even if consideration of a transplant candidate's criminal past is not allowed, it is likely that ex-prisoners will still be less likely to be accepted on waiting lists, because they are more likely to be poor, uninsured, and in general have less access to the medical care that might facilitate their receiving a transplant.

PHYSICIAN BEHAVIOR AND THE ORGAN WAITING LIST

One of the factors that influences priority for donor organs is medical necessity—people in the most critical condition, related to the organ for which they are waiting, get higher priority (unless, of course, their health has deteriorated to the point where a transplant would not help them). Those who administer the waiting list do not have the capacity to send an impartial physician to examine each patient, so the decision of who has the greatest medical need must be determined through review of each patient's medical records. One factor in this decision is the treatments prescribed to the patient, because they are a good indication of how serious the person's medical condition is. While the specific criteria vary depending on the organ an individual is waiting for and the criteria as well as the length of wait change over time, a hypothetical case discussed by Matthew Movesian illustrates the kind of ethical dilemma possible in this system.

Movesian uses the example of a patient who needs a heart transplant. Individuals on the waiting list for a donor heart receive a "status," based on their medical condition, which helps establish their priority. For instance, suppose someone receiving a particular drug intravenously to help the heart function would be classified as Status 1, while a similar patient not receiving that drug would be a Status 2. Persons classified as Status 1 have a shorter median wait time than those classified as Status 2, because they are considered to have greater medical need for a transplant. To make things even more complicated, a person receiving a high dosage of the drug in question is classified as Status 1A, while those receiving a low dosage are Status 1B and the median waiting time is less for a Status 1A than for a Status 1B individual. These determinations make medical sense, but the situation is complicated by the fact that different physicians may prescribe different courses of treatment for patients in a similar condition, because there is a great deal of human judgment involved in medicine. However, the physician's choice can have a major influence on how long a patient waits for a transplant, and the status classification system encourages physicians to prescribe treatments that will give their patient the best chance to receive a donor organ sooner.

Every physician wants the best for their patients, and some have argued that a bit of gaming the system in order to improve a patient's chances for a donor organ is ethical. One argument likens it to individuals who forged documents during World War II to save the lives of Jewish individuals. However, there is a counter to this argument, which is that the supply of donor organs is limited and insufficient, so acting to increase a particular patient's chances of getting an organ quickly means that someone else, with equal or greater claim to that organ, must wait longer. In other words, there is no societal benefit to favoring one person over another. In addition, if people believe the system is being gamed to favor people with money and power, they might be discouraged from signing up to be organ donors, thus reducing the overall organ supply.

There is an additional complication in this case: if physicians believe that their peers are already gaming the system, they may feel that they must do likewise or their patients will suffer unfairly. This scenario is not just an abstract possibility: Movesian cites research suggesting that invasive medical procedures are overused in patients on the transplant waiting list and that medical practice has changed over time in response to changes in the waiting list criteria. Unfortunately, given the shortage of donor organs, there may be no way to establish waiting list criteria that cannot be gamed in some way.

CONTACTING THE DONOR FAMILY

Organ transplant recipients and their families often want to meet the family of the person of the organ donor to thank them and to let them know the benefits that the donation brought about. Similarly, the donor's family may desire to meet the recipient of the organ(s) of their loved one. There is no law prohibiting an organ recipient and the family of a donor from meeting, but there are laws protecting the confidentiality of medical information, including that of the organ donor and recipient. Organ procurement organizations (OPOs) have rules in place to protect the privacy of the donor's family and the recipient, and organ transplant centers may also have specific rules in place to maintain confidentiality. It's possible that either or both of the donor's family and the transplant recipient may prefer to remain anonymous, and their privacy desires should be respected.

The UNOS suggests that the best way to initiate contact with a donor family is through the transplant coordinator who handled an individual's transplant. It is possible for a transplant recipient to write a card or letter thanking them and telling them something about the recipient (e.g., life events since receiving the transplant), but the card or letter should be left unsigned and not include specific information such as the recipient's address or the name of the transplant surgeon. The card or letter should be placed in an unsealed envelope and then placed inside another envelope that includes the name of the recipient and the date of the transplant. The outer envelope and its contents should be mailed to the transplant center, which should forward it to the OPO.

Someone at the OPO should review the letter and then contact the donor family to see if they wished to receive it. If the answer is no, the OPO should inform the transplant center, who should inform the transplant recipient. If the answer is yes, the letter should be forwarded to the donor's family, who may or may not prefer to respond. If they choose to respond, they should do so through the OPO, who would then forward their card or letter to the recipient. This method of communication allows both parties to express their gratitude and interest while maintaining their confidentiality. If both parties indicate through the OPO that they wish to have contact with the other, the OPO can arrange for them to meet directly.

THE ETHICS OF XENOTRANSPLANTATION

Xenotransplantation refers in a general sense to transplanting organs from one species to another, such as from a pig or baboon to a human. A more precise definition from the U.S. Food & Drug Administration, the agency responsible for regulating xenotransplantation in the United States, assumes that the recipient is human, and the materials transplanted, implanted, or infused are either live cells, tissues, or organs from an animal or human cells, tissues, organs, or body fluids that have been in contact *ex vivo* (outside the body) with living animal cells, tissues, or organs. A primary force driving research into xenotransplantation today is the hope that it could help reduce the current unmet demand for human organs for transplantation.

A number of ethical issues are relevant to xenotransplantation. The first is a consideration of the rights of animals. The reason xenotransplantation can offer an essentially unlimited supply of organs, tissues, and cells for transplantation into humans is because animals can be bred specifically for that purpose and their bodies used for the benefit of people. Nearly everyone would consider it unethical to raise human beings for that purpose, an idea presented in fictional form in the dystopian science fiction novel *Never Let Me Go* by Kazuo Ishiguro, in which cloned children are raised exclusively for the purpose of harvesting their organs after they reach adulthood. Some individuals, including people who identify with the animal right movement, argue that treating animals as fundamentally different from human beings is immoral. Someone holding those beliefs would probably not accept a transplant from an animal, or that containing animal cells, but since these beliefs have not become mainstream, they are unlikely to lead to a prohibition on xenotransplantation, any more than they have resulted in legal bans on, for instance, using lab animals for research, consuming meat, or wearing leather.

Another issue for some people would be the specific animal used in xenotransplantation. Pigs have become the favored donor animal for some types of xenotransplantation, due to the success in engineering the donor pig to reduce the immune response of the human recipient to the donor organ. However, pigs are considered unclean by some religions, including Judaism and Islam; recipients who observe those religions might object to receiving a transplant from a pig or that contained any pig cells. They would certainly be free to refuse such a transplant, but their choices do not ethically prohibit others who have no such objections from receiving potentially lifesaving treatment. One ethical question is raised with regard to both those who object to transplantations from animals and those who object to pigs specifically—should those individuals be favored on waiting lists for human organs, because they can't avail themselves of these alternative forms of treatment? To this point, the answer to that question has been no—xenotransplantation is currently considered an alternative that may help some individuals, but their choice to reject that alternative does not have any impact on an individual's priority for an organ transplant.

One societal concern with xenotransplantation is the possibility of transmitting microorganisms such as viruses, bacteria, fungi, and parasites from animal to human. While this type of transmission could be unfortunate for the recipient, it would be even more serious for society at large if the microorganism mutated into a form in which it could infect other humans. This could lead to the creation of a "super bug" to which no humans have immunity and which could thus quickly infect large numbers of people. Medical history is full of examples of serious diseases, including AIDS and Ebola, that evolved so that they could be transmitted from animals to humans, and many strain types of influenza are believed to have originated in animals before becoming able to infect humans. A particular concern, since pigs are often the animal of choice for providing donor cells, tissues, and organs to humans, is the transmission of porcine endogenous retroviruses from pig to human.

In the future, it might be possible to raise pathogen-free pigs specifically for the purposes of xenotransplantation or to purify their cells, organs, or tissues before the transplant takes place. However, until there is a sure method to ensure that microorganisms are not passed from animal to human during a xenotransplant, anyone receiving such a transplant might need to agree in advance to an increased level of monitoring following the operation. They might also have to accept temporary quarantine or restriction on activities that would bring them in contact with other people, particularly those vulnerable to infection. Any such arrangement, however, requires balancing two sets of rights—those of an individual to lead their life freely and that of society to be protected from potentially deadly infections.

ETHICAL CONCERNS WITH PAID ORGAN DONATIONS

The sale and purchase of human organs is considered unethical and prohibited in most countries of the world. One exception is Iran, which has allowed donation of kidneys to people other than relatives since 1988 and has created a government-run system that compensates donors. Some physicians and ethicists believe that the success of the Iranian program indicates that Western countries, including the United States, should consider allowing paid organ donation. In support, they point out that many people in the United States die each year while waiting for a donated organ. This is a classical ethical dilemma, in which a decision must be made between two "wrongs." On the one hand, there is no question that people are dying from kidney disease who could be saved given our current level of medical knowledge, and our best efforts to increase voluntary organ donation have not solved this problem. In some countries, the shortage of organs has given rise to a black market in which an organ will go to whoever can pay for it, rather than to the person who needs it most. On the other hand, the idea of paying a living donor to give up one of his or her kidneys is repugnant to many people, and it could easily lead to a situation in which the poor would literally sell their bodies to the rich.

Bioethicists frequently have to make judgments and recommendations in cases where there are multiple competing "wrongs" or multiple competing "rights," and they have developed an ethical framework in which to examine such situations. In this case, the primary conflict is between two "wrongs." Four principles are frequently cited as fundamental to bioethics: autonomy, beneficence, nonmaleficence, and justice. Autonomy refers to the right of every individual to self-determination, including the right to accept or refuse medical care. Beneficence refers to the obligation of medical professionals to act in their patient's best interest, while nonmaleficence refers to the corresponding obligation to avoid harming a patient. In the case where these principles come into conflict, for instance if surgery or other treatment might save a patient's life, but also carries some risk of harm or death, the guiding principle is that the decision should be made so that the expected benefits to the patient outweigh the potential harm.

The principle of justice is the most complicated, because there are several competing systems of justice that could be applied to the relationship between a patient and those providing him or her with medical care. Two leading philosophical systems of justice are that of utilitarianism, which focuses on utility or efficiency, and principles-based justice; a principles-based justice system guided by the principle of egalitarianism, for instance, would focus on distributing resources fairly. The two systems may come into conflict because a utilitarian system would distribute resources, including donor organs, in order to maximize lives saved or the number of life-years gained, while an egalitarian system might reduce efficiency as defined by these terms in order to create greater equity in the distribution of resources. In practice, the principles of both efficiency and equity are usually considered in the context of organ allocation, although different systems may give different emphasis to each: for instance, a system based in equity might value time spent on the waiting list more highly than a utilitarian system, while a utilitarian system might place greater emphasis on finding the best match between a donor and recipient.

Benjamin Hippen and colleagues use these principles of bioethics to examine the hypothetical case of the U.S. Senate holding a hearing on a bill that would allow payments of up to $10,000, plus reimbursement for expenses, to individuals willing to be living kidney, lung, or liver donors (there is currently no such law in the United States, although a similar bill was introduced in the Senate in 2008). At the hearing, the case is presented of a young woman suffering from end-stage renal disease who has had several dangerous bloodstream infections. No suitable donor is available within her family, and although she is wait-listed for a donor kidney, it is likely that she will die before receiving a kidney in that way. Her father has located several potential living donors from outside the family, but all are concerned about lost income, the possibility of losing their jobs, and the pain and physical risks of the operation. The father believes that if it were possible to provide a cash payment, income tax credit, and/or guarantee of health insurance following the donation, one of the potential donors might agree to donate a kidney and save his daughter's life.

The primary argument for allowing paid living organ donations is the shortage of donor organs and the corresponding number of people who experience a diminished quality of life while waiting for an organ and may ultimately die without receiving one. Despite loosening of the rules concerning who may donate an organ, and many campaigns to increase organ donation, the discrepancy between the number of donor organs needed, and the number available, continues to increase, and that pattern is expected to continue in the future.

An ethicist can appeal to the principle of autonomy to support financial incentives, including payment, for living organ donations. In a free society, individuals are generally allowed to make decisions for themselves, as long as those decisions do not harm others (or, possibly, do not harm themselves). However, in most countries, an individual is not allowed to make the decision to accept compensation in return for donating an organ, and this prohibition could be seen as an infringement on the rights of the individual.

Another argument in favor of allowing some kind of regulated incentives system for living donation is beneficence, in particular the benefits to be received and the harms to be alleviated by this choice. If the pool of donor organs was significantly expanded, as would be expected if compensation for donation was allowed, there would be reduced demand for organs obtained on the black market, and thus a reduction in organ trafficking. This in turn would reduce harm to individuals, generally poor people in poor countries, who risk their health in order to donate an organ or who are coerced into donating. Bringing payment for donated organs under government control and regulation should also reduce the risk to potential donors, because the donation and aftercare would take place in a hospital and treatment would be provided by qualified professionals. Increasing the pool of potential donors would also allow medical screening of donor candidates, with organs accepted from those least likely to be harmed by the process.

Any system of payment for organ donation would require regulation and oversight, and if the process was legal, it would be easier to prevent harm and maximize benefit. Among the principles by which such oversight should be provided are safety, transparency, institutional integrity, and the rule of law. The safety of both the donor and the recipient should be of primary concern, and it is more easily assured in a system that is legal and conducted within the normal health care system of a country. Transparency means that the process should be clear to both donors and recipients, and both should be fully aware of the risks involved in organ donation and transplantation. Institutional integrity means that everyone involved in the process should be free to establish their own moral and ethical principles and make their own decisions in accordance with those principles, including making the choice to take part in paid donation or not. The role of the rule of law in an organ donation system is to create a system of rules under which organ donation for mutual benefit would be allowed. Following these principles differentiates a legal system of organ donation for payment from organ trafficking.

Hippen and colleagues cite the success of the Iranian paid-donation system as evidence that a paid system could also work in the United States. They say that available evidence indicates that Iran has not had a waiting list for kidney transplants since at least 1996, a clear benefit given the number of people who die waiting for a kidney in the United States. They cite evidence that the long-term health outcomes for recipients of purchased as opposed to kidneys from unpaid donors are equivalent, indicating that the benefit of receiving a transplant is not offset by any evident harm if the kidney came from a paid donor.

An ethical argument can also be made that paid organ donations should not be allowed, demonstrating that ethical decisions are complex and depend on interpretation as well as how much weight is granted to different conflicting principles, benefits, or harms, in particular cases.

First, the argument against paid donations notes that the principle of autonomy is subject to moral constraints and exists within a social context. In the United States, for instance, we do not allow people to sell themselves into slavery, even if they claim they want to do so. Even those who are in favor of living kidney donation are likely to find a market in which a person could volunteer to kill themselves objectionable, donating all their organs in the process, with the resulting payments going to their family. An argument can be made that donating a kidney harms the individual, and the principle of autonomy does not preclude the challenging of individual decisions that are not in the individual's best interest. An argument can also be made that creating a market in which organs may be sold is degrading to the entire society, even if the market is conducted fairly. Medical personnel will necessarily be involved in the sale and receipt of human organs under such a system, and such participation could be seen as requiring them, against their professional principles, to harm one individual for the benefit of another.

The above objections apply to an idealized organ market, in which everyone involved is well informed and no one is coerced to take part in it. In reality, given the high levels of inequality in both income and political power in many parts of the world, it is entirely reasonable to assume that a paid system would be likely to result in the exploitation of the poor and powerless for the benefit of the rich and powerful. There is some evidence that in Iran donors are more likely to come from the poorest and least educated sectors of society and the recipients from the richest and the most educated. If the system allowed purchase of organs from non-U.S. donors, this risk would be even greater, because any amount in U.S. dollars has considerably more value in some countries (e.g., China, India) than it does in the United States. Creation of a legal market for donor organs in Iran has also not eradicated the black market, which is perhaps not surprising since legal and illegal markets can operate side by side. Despite laws prohibiting direct contact between potential donors and recipients, and contracting and paying for organs outside the official system, there are reports of young men visiting dialysis clinics and making it known that they have a "spare" kidney that could be donated.

Organ transplantation, while a lifesaving process, raises many ethical concerns. The dominant problem in organ transplantation is the shortage of donor organs, which therefore have to be allocated based on some system of priorities. While the purpose of an allocation system is to be fair to everyone, it is natural that some people might think that it favors one person or group of people over another or that physicians might be manipulating the system to favor their own patients. Some people find the concept of "brain death" confusing and concerning, but should be reassured to learn that they are strict, objective standards for declaring an individual brain dead and the fact of having registered as an organ donor is never allowed to influence the care a patient receives. It is natural for an organ recipient to want to meet the family of the person who donated their organ(s), but this process is best carried out through an organ procurement organization, in order to protect the privacy of everyone involved. While xenotransplantation may prove an excellent source for donor organs, it carries its own ethical concerns, including the possibility of engendering the creation of infectious "super bugs" that could spread to the population at large. Finally, the practice of paid human organ donation, which is legal in Iran, raises a number of ethical issues, and there are arguments both for and against permitting this type of organ donation.

PART III

Scenarios

CHAPTER 11

Case Studies

CASE 1: MICHAEL CONSIDERS BECOMING A LIVING ORGAN DONOR FOR HIS NEPHEW

Michael is a 32-year-old man who is married and has two preschool children, ages 2 and 4. He lives with his family in suburban Phoenix. Michael has one adult sibling, a brother, who has three children. One of those children, Michael's nephew, age 6, is suffering from a malignant liver tumor, and the brother's family has been informed that the child needs a liver transplant. Because of the shortage of suitable organs for transplant, the family has been advised to consider a living-related donor transplant. Michael's brother and his family live in Philadelphia, and due to the geographic distance between them, as well as both being busy establishing their careers and taking care of their families, Michael and his brother have not remained in close contact with each other. In fact, Michael was not aware of his nephew's illness until he was contacted about being screened as a potential living donor for the child.

Michael has always been healthy, and in fact, the only time he's been in a hospital was to visit his wife while their children were being born. He does not get annual medical checkups, and up to this point, he has never had an occasion to think much about either good health or disease. His wife and children have also been healthy, and his wife has always organized medical care for the children, scheduling their immunizations, checkups, and so on and taking them to appointments. Michael is not well informed on medical issues, such as the function of the liver within the body, the ability of the liver to regenerate, and the consequences of a poorly functioning liver. He is also not particularly up-to-date regarding advances made in medical care or the number of successful organ transplants performed annually.

The main reason Michael is aware of organ transplantation at all stems largely from news stories emphasizing the "miraculous" nature of organ transplantation and human-interest stories about individuals whose lives were saved due to their receiving an organ transplant. Often these stories are meant to encourage organ donation, but the organs nearly always come from a deceased donor, so he's not sure how such stories relate to the possibility of a living person donating part of an organ. In fact, to him the latter process seems like something a mad scientist in a science fiction movie might attempt, and he finds the idea of taking part in such an operation uncomfortable and off-putting.

However, because Michael loves his brother and his nephew and sincerely wants to help them, he agrees to undergo screening to see if he is a suitable donor. At the same time, he begins reading about organ transplantation in general, and living organ donation in particular, so that he will be better informed if the time comes that he must decide whether he wants to donate part of his liver to his nephew or not. He does not like the idea of voluntarily going to the hospital to have an operation and is concerned about the possibilities of suffering complications from the surgery, or from living with a partial liver, which might impair his ability to care for his own family. Although he is reluctant to mention it, Michael is also worried that the process of living with a partial liver would mean that he is less "whole" or "complete" than before the surgery.

Michael has been informed that he is a match for his nephew and has agreed to meet with a psychologist familiar with organ transplant issues to better inform himself about the process and to help himself decide if he wants to become a living donor or not. Michael's brother is upper middle class and has agreed to cover any expenses Michael incurs that are not covered by insurance, including lost wages if he is unable to work for a period of time following the surgery.

Analysis

What role does a transplant psychologist play in the process of organ donation and transplantation? A transplant psychologist in an individual who has earned a PhD degree in psychology and who has chosen to specialize in working with people involved in organ donation and transplantation, receiving specialized training in these issues. Although not an MD, the transplant psychologist has a good understanding of the transplant process from a nontechnical point of view and is skilled in communicating medical information to people who are neither physicians nor scientists. This psychologist has a lot of experience in educating potential donors and recipients about the donation and transplant process as well as evaluating their psychological condition, helping them clarify their thoughts and feelings, and helping them work through any mental or emotional problems they may be experiencing. The purpose of Michael's meeting with this psychologist is not to influence him toward making any particular decision, but to educate him on the facts regarding living donation and help him think through any concerns he may have and then make an informed decision that is right for him.

Michael has conflicting feelings about being a living organ donor. He is sure that he wants to help his nephew if he can, but is also feeling that he doesn't well understand the process of living donation. In addition, he feels his first obligation is to take care of his own family and is concerned about the possible adverse impacts on himself and his own family were he to donate part of his liver. The first thing the psychologist can do is help Michael understand the nephew's medical condition, why he needs a liver transplant and why a living donation is his best option. Topics he will bring up in this discussion include the shortage of donor organs from deceased donors and the improved outcomes, including shorter recovery times, typical when a transplanted liver comes from a living donor. He can also help Michael understand the importance of the liver within the human body and the unusual ability it has to regenerate itself. Because the nephew's body is much smaller than that of an adult, a partial liver from an adult donor will function normally in the nephew's body and will grow along with the rest of his body to become a complete organ. Equally important, Michael will have only a partial liver following the transplant, but it will regenerate within his body so that he will once again have a complete liver.

The psychologist can also explain to Michael that if he chooses to become a living donor, he will have to undergo some inconvenience and discomfort, but it is unlikely he will experience any serious medical complications. Hospitals have been performing living-donor donation for decades and are well prepared to deal with any of the complications that may ensue, including infection, bleeding, and blood clots. The psychologist will listen to Michael's concerns and help him clarify his thoughts and feelings, without trying to direct his decision-making process. If Michael is interested, the psychologist can also put Michael in touch with a living donor who has consented to share his experiences regarding the process.

CASE 2: MARIA LEARNS ABOUT THE PROCESS OF BECOMING A HEART TRANSPLANT RECIPIENT

Maria is a 23-year-old woman living in New York City. She is not married and works long hours as a financial consultant for a company in the city. She recently suffered a viral infection that resulted in heart damage. This turn of events came as a shock to her, because, prior to her illness, she had had no significant health issues: in fact, she had been a scholarship athlete in college and continued to swim and play tennis recreationally after graduation. She has always been a high achiever and enjoys setting difficult challenges for herself and then meeting them. This process and the resulting success gave the sense that she was in control of her life and that she could accomplish anything she set out to do. The illness and resulting heart damage are the first serious setbacks she has experienced in her life, and although she has recovered well enough to return to work, she has recently been informed by her physician that her best chance for long-term survival is a heart transplant.

Maria has good health insurance through her job. Although Maria lives with a roommate in a condo in the city, her family home is less than an hour's drive away, and she has maintained a close relationship with her parents. Although she makes her own decisions regarding her health, her family is willing to provide whatever support she needs, and she has the option of returning to the family home should her health require it. Maria's parents are concerned for their daughter's health, of course, but are also aware that she faces emotional and psychological challenges as a result of her illness and the inevitable waiting and uncertainty inherent in the organ allocation process. Maria is used to thinking of herself as the master of her own fate, so they are concerned that the prospect of having to wait for an outcome that is not assured, and that which she can do little to influence, is likely to pose a serious challenge to her sense of self.

Maria's physician has given her a referral, and she has begun the process of registering for the waiting list at a transplant hospital recommended by her physician. In fact, she has already completed some of the physical screening tests, and so far remains eligible to receive a transplant. Her next appointment is with a transplant counselor who will describe how the transplant waiting list functions and will answer any questions she has about the process and refer her to further sources of information or support as necessary.

Analysis

Maria is fortunate in many ways—she has good health insurance and sufficient financial resources to manage the expenses involved in organ transplantation, she has a supportive family close at hand, and she lives in an urban area noted for the availability of advanced health care, including the presence of multiple transplant hospitals. The latter means that she has the option of multiple listing, meaning adding herself to the waiting list at more than one transplant hospital; this practice, although somewhat controversial, might improve her chances of receiving a donated heart. Although she doesn't know much about how the organ donation, allocation, and transplantation system works, she is ready to do whatever she can to improve her chances of survival.

The first thing the transplant counselor can do is give Maria some basic information about the process she is beginning, including what she can expect in the upcoming months and years. Her heart has suffered sufficient damage that, in the opinion of her physician, it will need to be replaced by a donor heart at some time in the foreseeable future. Like many transplant procedures, heart transplantation was an experimental procedure when it was first developed in the 1960s, but is now an established form of treatment, with over 2,000 heart transplants performed in the United States annually. While the survival time following a transplant is influenced by many factors, some people have lived for decades following a heart transplant. Due to a shortage of donor organs, Maria's name will be added to a waiting list, where her priority for a donor heart will be based on a number of factors, including her health status and the availability of donor hearts within her region.

The counselor can help Maria understand her current situation and acknowledge that it is a major and unexpected disruption, introducing uncertainty at a time when she seemed to be on course for a long and successful life. She can also let Maria know that other young adults have received heart transplants, found it to be a largely positive experience, and have led fruitful posttransplant lives. The counselor can also help Maria accept the fact that while she can't directly influence her priority for receiving a donor heart (or even the availability of a suitable donor heart), there are certain things she can do to ensure that, if a donor organ becomes available, she will still be eligible to receive it.

The first thing Maria needs to do while on the waiting list is to keep all her appointments and comply with all the regulations of the transplant center, as well as the recommendation of her primary physician. Living successfully with a transplanted organ requires following a strict regime, and she needs to indicate through her behavior that she would be willing and able to do so should she have the opportunity of receiving a donor heart. The second thing Maria can do is to keep herself as healthy as possible, both psychologically and physically, so that she is not later disqualified from receiving an organ for mental or physical reasons. She needs to use the resources available to her to cope with the stress of waiting for a transplant and in particular to avoid behaviors that could disqualify her, such as self-harm and substance abuse. Finally, the counselor can refer Maria to further psychological and other resources to help her cope with the inevitable stress of waiting for a donor organ.

CASE 3: JOSH CONSIDERS MEDICAL TOURISM AS A MEANS TO OBTAIN A DONOR KIDNEY

Josh is a 50-year-old man who is divorced and has two adult children who live in other parts of the country, so he does not see them regularly. He has spent most of his career working as a computer programmer, a job that provided him with excellent health insurance as well as allowing him to save for retirement. He enjoyed his work and took an important part of his identity from his professional success and the role he played in his company. His job also provided him with a structure to his life, as well as regular contact with other people—in fact, most of the people he socializes with are people he also works with. Josh and his wife attended the Methodist Church when their children were young, because they wanted them to have some experience of religion, but since the divorce and the children moving out of the house, Josh has not attended any kind of religious service.

Josh has suffered from chronic kidney disease for some years, but has been able to keep working until fairly recently. About six months ago, Josh's physician informed him that his eGFR (estimated glomerular filtration rate, a measurement of kidney function) had dropped below 15. This means that he has less than 15% of normal kidney function, which classifies him as having stage five kidney disease and kidney failure. Josh began hemodialysis and tried to keep working part-time, but found that it was too difficult, so he took early retirement and switched his insurance coverage to Medicare (having kidney failure and being on dialysis qualifies an individual for Medicare coverage, regardless of age).

Josh resents the fact that his life is now structured around going to his dialysis appointments (he receives four-hour treatments three times a week). He also dislikes being dependent on what he feels is invasive medical treatment and has had difficulty in following the dietary guidelines his physician has provided. For instance, he has always enjoyed salty snacks, which he must now avoid, and does not fully understand why he has been told to avoid some foods that he thinks of as healthy, such as orange juice, bananas, and yoghurt. Finally, he finds the limits on fluid intake (32 ounces per day) to be particularly difficult to follow and has suffered from fluid overload.

Josh also mourns the loss of his ability to work. His days feel unstructured and pointless apart from his dialysis treatments, and he misses seeing his coworkers every day. While he has made some attempts to stay in touch with his former office buddies, he now feels out of sync with them. In addition, the dietary and fluid restrictions he must follow make activities like going to a sports bar, which he used to do regularly with friends from work, more of a chore than a pleasure.

Josh is not looking forward to spending the rest of his life on dialysis, and he has also heard that his life expectancy would be longer if he received a kidney transplant. He is registered on a waiting list to receive a donor kidney, but is aware that there are not enough donor kidneys in the United States for everyone who needs one and that he might die on the waiting list. For these reasons, he is considering traveling to another country to receive a kidney transplant. He has enough money saved to pay for the travel and the transplant, but is concerned about the safety of the process and also whether Medicare will cover his aftercare expenses when he returns to the United States. He has raised the possibility of obtaining a kidney transplant through medical tourism with his personal physician.

Analysis

The physician needs to help Josh with two types of issues. The first are measures Josh can take to improve his health and quality of life while continuing to receive dialysis. The second are issues regarding medical tourism that Josh needs to educate himself about, before deciding if that is the best course of action for him. The physician can begin by reassuring Josh that it is not unusual for a patient to have difficulties adapting to the process of dialysis, including the dietary restrictions that must be followed. He can explain more about how dialysis works and why it is necessary—that dialysis removes waste, salt, and excess water from his body, helps control his blood pressure, and controls the level of certain chemicals in his body, all functions his kidneys can no longer perform effectively—and can remind Josh that he would not be expected to live for long were he to stop dialysis treatment.

The physicians can also make several referrals to help Josh. One could be to a counselor who works with dialysis patients and can help Josh settle into the treatment regime and adjust to the fact that his life is now dependent on receiving regular dialysis treatment. The counselor can help Josh look at his current life and determine what changes he would like to make and develop a plan to meet any goals he wants to set. For instance, it might be possible for Josh to return to work part-time once he adjusts to the dialysis process, and he can also take steps to meet people not connected with his workplace.

The physician can refer Josh to a nutritionist, who can help him understand why the dietary restrictions are important, give him meal plans and recipes that are healthy for him, and suggest ways he can substitute different foods for those that are restricted. One example would be to cook using a variety of permitted spices rather than salt, so his food tastes good but he doesn't exceed the guidelines for sodium intake. Finally, the physician can refer Josh to a support group of other dialysis patients. This will both help him break out of his current social isolation and give him a chance to find out how other people have dealt with the issues he is now facing.

If, after taking these steps, Josh decides he wants to pursue a kidney transplant through medical tourism, the physician can advise him to carefully research the process. In a country other than the United States, the standards of care may be different from what Josh expects, and physicians will not be bound by American laws or customs. Josh also needs to think carefully about how he feels, from an ethical point of view, about purchasing the kidney of a living person and whether that means he is exploiting someone else's poverty. To aid in this process, the physician can suggest he talk to a minister at his former church. If Josh prefers, the physician can refer him to a counselor familiar with ethical issues regarding organ transplants. The physician can also suggest that Josh speak to others in the support group, and to someone at the transplant center where he is registered, to see what they may know about the process. He can also point out that Medicare will not pay for transplant expenses overseas, but will pay for aftercare in the United States.

CASE 4: PATRICIA RECOVERS FOLLOWING A CORNEAL TRANSPLANT

Patricia is a 35-year-old woman who teaches high school English in suburban Atlanta. She began having symptoms of keratoconus, including blurred vision and sensitivity to bright lights, when she was in her twenties. Keratoconus is caused by a change in the shape of the cornea, the dome-shaped outer surface of the eye, in which the cornea becomes thinner and bulges into a cone shape; this change in shape causes distortions in vision. Initially, Patricia wore glasses to correct her vision and then switched to rigid contact lenses. Unfortunately, Patricia's disease continued to progress and her visual difficulties worsened, eventually making it difficult for her to work and to carry out activities of normal life, such as shopping (the bright lights in stores became painful to her). Due to the increasing impairment caused by her condition, Patricia's ophthalmologist suggested she consider receiving a corneal transplant, a procedure also known as keratoplasty, in which her damaged corneal tissue would be removed surgically and replaced with healthy corneal tissue from a deceased human donor.

Patricia was surprised at this advice, because she associated corneal transplants with elderly people (one of her grandmothers had had a corneal transplant, for instance, and was pleased with the results). But after reading more about the subject and consulting several specialists, she decided that a corneal transplant would be the best course of action for her. Because corneal transplants are performed one eye at a time, she was relieved to know that she would have one "good" eye to see out of while the other eye was healing.

Investigating the process of corneal transplant, Patricia was surprised to learn that she did not have to be placed on a waiting list, because there is not the same shortage for corneas as for most organs. The cornea is a body tissue, not an organ, and many of the complications of organ transplants do not apply to corneal transplants. For instance, because the cornea does not contain blood vessels, the donor and recipient do not have to have the same blood type. In addition, nearly everyone can donate their corneas after death (there are only a few disqualifying conditions, although one requirement is that the donor cornea is an appropriate size for the recipient), and donor corneas can be kept in a suitable state for transplant for up to 14 days. For these reasons, corneal transplant operations are normally scheduled in advance, although the date of the surgery might be moved up if a suitable donor cornea becomes available or delayed if a suitable donor cornea is not available at the scheduled time. Patricia was also gratified to learn that corneal transplant has a high success rate (figures as high as 95% and 97% have been reported in different sources).

Patricia had her corneal transplant done as an outpatient procedure, as is the norm, and returned home the same day. Her left eye was operated on first, and she experienced no discomfort during the surgery. Following some recovery time under observation at the clinic, she returned home the same day. Because she had been told she would not be able to drive the same day of the surgery, due to the drugs used during the surgery, she arranged for a friend to drive her home. She received eyedrops to suppress the immune system and help prevent rejection, and she was expected to continue to do so for at least a year.

The transplant was covered by her insurance, and Patricia was able to use sick leave time from her job to stay home for a few days. While the operation went well, Patricia was disappointed to find that she was still suffering from blurred version in her left eye two weeks after the transplant; she had expected quicker improvement in her vision. The blurred vision was interfering with her desires to resume her normal life: she did not feel safe driving while only one eye was functioning normally, for instance, which was a real problem since there was little public transportation where she lived. Overall, she felt that she was not sufficiently informed about what the recovery process would entail. She has made an appointment with an ophthalmologist (not the one she usually sees) to learn more about what to expect in the upcoming weeks and months.

Analysis

The ophthalmologist can begin by clarifying to Patricia that although corneal transplant has an extremely high success rate, that does not mean that the eye receiving the donor cornea will immediately function like a normal eye. Her symptoms are completely normal for someone who has just had a corneal transplant and are not indicative of a failed procedure or rejection. In particular, it is normal for the recipient's vision to be worse than before immediately after the surgery, and it is not uncommon for it to take several months before vision in the transplanted eye improves substantially. She also tells Patricia that her vision will likely improve in stages and that adjustments can be made to her cornea after the outer layer has healed. For instance, the stiches holding the donor cornea in place might be causing her blurry vision. Once the outer layer of the cornea has healed, an ophthalmologist can perform procedures that might improve her vision, such as removing some of the stiches or tightening some of them. Patricia might also need a different prescription for her glasses or contact lenses when her eye has healed.

She can also let Patricia know that she is doing the right thing by seeking out further information and emphasize the importance of following all the directions given to her by the surgeon. These instructions include using eye drops for at least a year to suppress the immune system and prevent rejection, wearing an eye shield to protect the transplanted eye while it heals, and taking it easy for the days after surgery. She also noted that Patricia would always need to protect the transplanted eye from injury and would need to return to her regular ophthalmologist regularly for follow-up appointments, particularly in the first year after her surgery, and to plan on annual eye exams after that time (all of this medical care is covered by Patricia's employer-based health insurance). Finally, she can emphasize to Patricia that most corneal transplant recipients eventually experience improved vision and that she should think of the recovery process as just that—a process that she needs to go through to get the improved vision that she seeks.

CASE 5: JOSE'S FAMILY CONSIDERS DONATING HIS ORGANS

Jose, an 18-year-old college student living with his parents in Los Angeles, is an avid motorcyclist. Unfortunately, he was in a serious road accident and has been brought to the emergency department of a hospital that includes a Level I Trauma Center. The medical staff determines that he has suffered a severe traumatic brain injury (TBI) along with other serious physical injuries. Despite receiving the best possible medical care, the blood supply to his brain ceased for a sufficient period of time such that he is brain dead. One of the hospital physicians performs the necessary tests and diagnoses Jose as brain dead; a second physician at the hospital confirms the diagnosis, and Jose is declared legally dead. He has not registered as an organ donor and neither has anyone else in his immediate family.

Jose comes from a large, close-knit Catholic family. When his parents hear that he has been in an accident, they rush to the hospital, and they have received regular updates from the medical staff on his condition. They trust the medical staff to deliver the best possible care to their son, but are not familiar with medical terminology and are confused by the term "brain dead." They don't understand how there could be different types of death and don't see why their son would be determined to be dead if his body was showing any signs of life, nor why the hospital has placed him on a ventilator if he is truly dead. There is something of a communication barrier because their first language is Spanish, although they also speak and understand English.

Jose's parents are even more confused when a transplant counselor working for the hospital approaches them to broach the subject of donating their son's organs. Although the counselor is compassionate and professional, Jose's parents are grieving due to their son's accident and are not sure that they want to talk to someone who seems to have a motivation that might not lead to the best outcome for him. They find it odd that they are being approached by a hospital employee about donating their son's organs when, by their way of thinking, he may well recover. In fact, the whole process seems a bit ghoulish to them, although they are more confused than angry. They fear that if they consider donating his organs, the hospital may no longer try to save his life and might even hasten his death.

Analysis

The organ donation counselor is a key member of the organ donation and transplant system. In this case, the counselor is an RN who has received specialized training as a designated requestor (someone who approaches families about organ donation) and has been working in her current position for five years. She has spoken to many grieving families and is always tactful and considerate, beginning the discussion by sharing her understanding of their shock and grief. In the case of Jose's parents, because they have identified themselves as Catholics, she lets them know that the hospital has a Catholic priest available if they would like to speak with him. She also lets them know that the hospital has bilingual English-Spanish translators who can be called in to help with communication. She assures Jose's parents that any decisions about their son will be made by them, that she understands this is a difficult time for them, and that she is not here to try to pressure them in any way. The counselor can also assure Jose's parents that he is not suffering and that the hospital did everything possible to save his life.

The counselor can explain what "brain death" means, since many people find the term confusing. A person who is brain dead is dead, and cannot be revived, because the damage to the brain is irreversible. Brain death is different from coma, because a person in a coma still has brain activity and function, while there is no brain function in the case of brain death. The process of declaring a person brain dead requires a series of specific tests, based on legally accepted medical guidelines, which are performed by a physician and in this hospital must also be confirmed by a second physician. While the patient is undergoing the tests to determine if brain death has occurred, he or she is placed on a ventilator so the body continues to receive oxygen; the ventilator is necessary because the brain is no longer able to send the necessary signals to the body that would enable the patient to breathe on their own. Because the patient's body is receiving oxygen, his or her heart continues to beat; were the ventilator to be withdrawn, the heart would stop beating.

The counselor can also explain a bit about how the organ donation and transplantation system works. She can use her judgment about how much information to give the family at this time, but might mention that many lives can be saved through organ transplantation and that some families have found donation to play a useful role in helping them deal with their loved one's death. She can assure them that there will be no visible signs on their son's body due to the donation process, so they will be able to have an open-casket funeral for him if that is their preference. She can also emphasize that their son's body will be treated with the utmost care and respect during the organ donation process. Finally, she can emphasize that they do not have to make a decision immediately, that she is available to speak with them further, and she can offer once again to summon other hospital resources, including a translator and a priest, if they would like.

GLOSSARY

Actual deceased organ donor: A person who is deceased and for whom one or more organs have been recovered to be used in transplantation, whether it is actually used for that purpose or not.

Acute rejection: Rapid rejection of a donated organ, due to triggering of the body's natural immune response system. Acute rejection is usually defined as rejection that occurs within the first year after a transplant.

Advance directive: A statement, usually in writing, by an individual stating what actions should be taken regarding their health if they are unable to make or express decisions in this regard.

Adverse reaction: An unintended, negative side effect of a procedure or the administration of a drug.

Allocation: A system used to assign available donor organs, tissues, or other human material to individuals requiring a transplant. Many different allocation systems, governed by different principles, are used in different parts of the world. Organ allocation systems are necessary due in part to the shortage of available organs relative to the number of individuals needing a transplant.

Allogeneic: Cells from different individuals of the same species. An allogeneic transplant is the transplantation of organs, cells, or tissues donated by one person into the body of another person.

Amniotic membrane: The innermost layer of the placental membrane, which surrounds the fetus during pregnancy.

Antigen: A molecule, usually a protein, that is capable of triggering the body's immune response. The body produces proteins called antibodies in response to antigens.

Antirejection drugs: Also called immunosuppressive drugs, drugs taken by an organ recipient to reduce their body's normal response to reject and destroy the transplanted organ.

Approach rate: The percentage of potential donor families approached to authorize organ donation.

Ascites: A collection of fluid in the abdomen; ascites is sometimes a consequence of liver disease.

Autologous transplantation: The transplantation of cells or tissues within the body of a single person, for instance, to repair or replace damaged tissue. Autologous transplantation is used during some types of medical treatment that are known to destroy a patient's bone marrow. In this procedure, some of the patient's bone marrow is removed before treatment and transplanted back into the patient when the treatment is concluded.

Autoresuscitation: Spontaneous restoration of heart function after the heart has ceased to beat.

Bone marrow: Tissue present in the center of hollow bones, such as those in the leg, arm, and pelvis, which contains stem cells and where new blood cells are produced. Two types of stem cells are contained in the bone marrow: hematopoietic, which can produce blood cells, and stromal, which can produce fat, cartilage, and bone. The pelvic bone is usually the source for the bone marrow used in bone marrow transplants.

Brain death: Also known as brain stem death, brain death is defined as the absence of brain function and electrical activity in the brain, as assessed by a clinician, and the irreversible cessation of brain function. A person who is brain dead may have cardiopulmonary function, although they are legally dead, and may be referred to as a "heart-beating donor" if their cardiac system is still functioning.

Cannulation: The placement of cannulae (tubes) into large blood vessels for the administration of fluids or withdrawal of blood.

Cardiac death: Also known as circulatory death, cardiac death is defined by the irreversible cessation of respiratory and circulatory function.

Chronic rejection: Slow failure of a donated organ, due to triggering of the body's natural immune response system.

Clinical triggers: A set of clinical criteria that indicate a high probability of death and that indicate that a hospital should initiate referral for organ donation.

Cold ischemia time: The time between the removal of an organ from the donor and the time it is transplanted into the recipient. During cold ischemia time, the organ does not have blood circulation and is kept cold. Cold ischemia time can also refer to the time during which an organ is kept chilled, which may include some time when it is still in a deceased donor's body.

Cold perfusion: A method for preserving organs *in situ*, that is, within the body of a deceased donor, until they can be removed. Cold perfusion involves the infusion of cold preservative solution into the vessels and the draining of blood.

Compatibility testing: Testing for HLA and blood group antigens, for the purpose of determining if a transplant is possible, on the cells, tissues, or organ(s) to be transplanted.

Compliance: Following medical treatment as prescribed, including matters such as taking specific medications at designated times or performing physical exercises as directed.

Consent rate: The proportion of families of eligible donors who authorized organ donation after being formally approached for their authorization.

Conversion rate: The proportion of potential donors who give their consent to donate. The term "conversion rate" is also used to refer to the percentage of donors who become actual donors.

Cord blood: Blood collected from umbilical cord vessels and placental vessels, which can serve as a source of hematopoietic progenitor cells.

Cornea: The transparent tissue in the front of the eye, which covers the iris and pupil.

Corticosteroid: A hormone present in the body, but which can also be synthesized in the lab for use as a drug for various medical purposes, including suppressing the body's response to foreign tissue or for other medical purposes. Examples of synthetic corticosteroids include prednisone, fludrocortisone, and hydrocortisone.

Cross-matching: A type of blood test used to determine if a donor organ is likely to be rejected by the proposed recipient. A positive cross-matching test indicates incompatibility between organ and recipient, and under those conditions, a transplant is unlikely to be carried out.

Cryopreservation: Preservation and storage by freezing or vitrification, or at low temperature, of viable tissues and cells.

Deceased donor: A donor who is dead before his or her organs are donated; death may be indicated by either cardiac death or brain death.

Deceased heart-beating donor: A donor who has been declared dead due to brain death, but whose cardiac system is still functioning.

Deceased non-heart-beating donor: A donor who is declared dead due to cardiopulmonary criteria.

Delayed function: In the context of an organ transplant, delayed function refers to the situation when a donated organ does not begin to work as expected soon after the transplant is performed.

Designated requestor: In the United States, someone who has completed an approved course in the appropriate methods of approaching potential donor families and requesting that they approve organ donation.

Dialysis: A medical process used to correct fluid balance and remove wastes from the blood when a person's kidneys are not functioning correctly and thus cannot perform these tasks adequately. Two types of dialysis exist: hemodialysis and peritoneal dialysis.

Directed altruistic donor: An organ donor who provides one or more organs to a recipient they designed, but who is not related emotionally or genetically to the recipient.

Directive 2010/53/EU: The document establishing the legal framework for organ transplantation in the European Union. This directive includes quality and safety standards and covers all stages of the transplant process from procurement to distribution.

Domino donor: An organ donor who both receives an organ transplant and donates the removed organ to another recipient. Domino transplants can involve more than two people, but these cases are rare.

Donor: A person who contributes cells, tissues, or organs for transplantation to another person. A donor may be living or dead, and a person from whom organs are recovered for transplant is considered a donor whether or not the organ or organs in question were actually used for transplant.

Donor card: A pocket-sized card indicating an individual's wish to be an organ donor after their death. In the United States, the driver's license often serves as a donor card, carrying an indication of whether the individual is part of the state's organ donor registry or not.

Donor designation: Official documentation of a person's intention to donate their organs, tissues, etc. after death, often by becoming part of a registry. In the United States, donor designation is often visible on the individual's driver's license.

Donor pool: A group of people who are eligible to donate an organ.

Donor registry: A database that contains the official designations of individuals who wish to be organ and tissue donors. The arrangement of donor registries varies by country—for instance, in the United States, they are usually organized at the state level, while in other countries a single registry may exist for the entire country.

Eligible death: Death of a person who is eligible to donate their organs. The criteria for organ donor eligibility are regularly updated, but may include stipulations concerning age of death, absence of particular infectious diseases, body weight, body mass index, and presence of one or more specific organs that meet the qualifications for transplant.

Emotionally related donor: A donor who is not genetically related to a recipient, but has an emotional relationship with them, such as a spouse or friend.

End-stage organ disease: A disease that can be predicted to lead to complete failure of an organ, such as emphysema (which leads to lung failure), polycystic kidney disease, or cardiomyopathy (which leads to hear failure).

ESRD: End-stage renal disease, the complete or nearly complete failure of the kidneys to perform their usual functions.

Explicit consent: A legally valid statement that an individual gives permission for their organs, cells, etc. to be transplanted; explicit consent is required in an "opt-in" system of organ donation.

First Person Consent Legislation: Laws in some states and countries that allow organ procurement to proceed, if an individual has indicated their wishes for this to be conducted upon their death, without requiring the consent of the individual's family.

Fulminant: A disease or condition that begins suddenly or escalates quickly and is severe; the term comes from the Latin term meaning "to strike with lightning."

Genetically related donor: A donor who is genetically related to the recipient, such as a brother, sister, parent, or child.

Glomular filtration rate: A measure of the severity of kidney disease based on calculations regarding how well the kidneys are currently filtering the blood. The eGFR (expected glomular filtration rate) is used to determine stages of kidney functioning and to define kidney failure.

Graft survival: The period of time after transplant during which an organ functions successfully.

Graft survival rate: The proportion of patients who have received an organ transplant whose organ is functioning correctly, as determined at some point in time.

HCTT: Human cells and tissues for transplantation, a definition that includes musculoskeletal tissue, skin, soft tissue, cardiovascular tissue, ocular tissue, bone marrow, and hematopoietic stem and progenitor cells. Examples of materials not considered HCTTs include vascularized human organs for transplantation, whole blood, blood components, blood products, secreted or excreted human products, and material from nonhuman animals.

Hematopoietic progenitor cells (HPC): Also known as hematopoietic stem cells, primitive hematopoietic cells that can both self-renew and can mature into any of the hematopoietic lineages.

Hemodialysis: A treatment in which a patient's blood is passed through a filter to remove excess fluid and wastes; hemodialysis is used to treat patients whose kidneys have failed.

Heparin: A medication that prevents blood clotting and is used in the organ donation process to maximize blood flow by keeping the blood vessels open.

Hepatitis: A disease marked by inflammation of the liver, which can lead to liver failure.

Histocompatibility: Also called tissue typing, the process of testing for antigens to see if a donor organ will be accepted by the potential recipient's body.

HLA: Human Leukocyte Antigens, a series of markers on human white blood cells and body tissues. HLAs are genetically determined, and matching for HLAs is an important step in assessing the compatibility of organs and recipients.

Human Tissue Authority: The organization regulating human tissue and organ donation in the United Kingdom, including living and deceased organ donation and entire body donation.

Idiopathic: An adjective meaning "of unknown origin," which is used to refer to a disease or condition that attacks an organ but the cause or mechanism of which is not known.

Immune response: The natural response of the human body against foreign organisms and objects. The immune response is useful when it identifies and attacks bacteria that has infected the body, but poses a problem in organ transplantation, because the body's natural response is to attack the transplanted organ.

Immunosuppressive drugs: Also called antirejection drugs, immunosuppressive drugs are used to suppress the body's natural immune response, which is to attack foreign objects such as transplanted organs. Immunosuppressive drugs play a key role in the success of organ transplants today. Examples of immunosuppressive drugs include cyclosporine, prednisone, and azathioprine.

Informed consent: Consent given voluntarily and based on complete and accurate information regarding what the person is consenting to. Informed consent is a standard requirement for many medical procedures and for participation in medical research.

Ischemia: A lack of oxygen supplied to the organs and tissues. Ischemia may either be warm, meaning that the heart and lungs are functioning but not adequately, or cold, which occurs after organs are removed from the body.

Kidneys: Organs involved in the process of maintaining water and electrolyte balance, filtering metabolic waste, and regulating acid-base concentration.

Lasting Power of Attorney (LPA): A legal document that indicates that an adult has chosen another person to make decisions on their behalf, including decisions about their health and welfare.

Leukocyte: Commonly called "white blood cells," leukocytes are made in the bone marrow and circulate in the blood and lymph tissue. Leukocytes are part of the body's immune system and help to fight infection.

Liver: An organ that performs several important bodily functions, including forming blood proteins, metabolizing carbohydrates, fats, and protein, and assists in removing toxins and wastes from the blood stream. Unlike many organs, the liver can regenerate, so it is possible for a partial liver to be transplanted successfully, and then both partial livers (in the donor's and recipient's bodies) can grow to become complete livers.

Living donor: A living person who has donated organs, cells, or tissues to another person. Living donors are classified as related or unrelated. Within those categories, a related donor may be genetically related (e.g., a sibling, parent, or child) or emotionally related (e.g., a spouse or friend), while an unrelated donor may be paired, nondirected altruistic, or directed altruistic.

Lungs: Body organs that allow the inhalation of air, provide oxygen to the body, and allow the exhalation of carbon dioxide. In some cases, a recipient may be helped by transplantation of a single lung or part of a lung, in which case a living donor may be used.

Lymphocytotoxic Crossmatch Test: A test that detects antibodies in the recipient that might react with HLA antigens from a donated organ. A positive lymphocytotoxic crossmatch test means that rejection of a donated organ is likely, and therefore, the transplant is unlikely to proceed.

Maastricht categories: Categories developed in 1995 to classify non-beating-heart donors. Category I refers to individuals who were dead upon arrival; Category II refers to those for whom attempts at resuscitation were unsuccessful; Category II refers to those awaiting cardiac arrest; Category IV refers to those suffering cardiac arrest after brain stem death; and Category V refers to cardiac arrest in a hospital patient.

Match: The degree of compatibility between an organ and a potential recipient.

Match run: A list generated when information from an organ donor is entered into a computer system containing the waiting list for potential recipients. The purpose of a match run is to identify potential recipients of the donor's organs.

National Organ Transplant Act (NOTA): An American law, passed in 1984, which began the development of a national system of organ sharing and a registry to collect scientific data related to transplants. NOTA also outlawed the sale of human organs in the United States.

Next of kin: An individual's closest living blood relative.

Nominated representative: A person chosen by an organ donor to represent the interests of the donor after the donor's death.

Noncompliance: Failure to follow medical instruction, for instance, not taking prescribed medications.

Nondirected donor: An organ donor who provides one or more organs for transplant but does not specify to whom they should go.

Organ: A differentiated structure of tissues in a human being or other living organism that performs a particular function; examples or organs include the heart, lungs, and kidneys. Organs are made up of similar types of tissue, and organs may combine to form organ systems, such as the respiratory system or the cardiovascular system.

Organ Procurement and Transplantation Network (OPTN): A network created in the United States in 1984 through the National Organ Transplant Act, with the purpose of improving the national procurement, donation, and transplantation system.

Organ Procurement Organizations (OPO): Organizations in the United States that play key roles in the organ donation process, including recruiting and registering donors and coordinating the donation process.

Organ yield metric: A statistic computed by dividing the observed number of organs transplanted by the expected number of organs transplanted. The expected number of organs transplanted in this statistic is an estimate based on national experience with similar donors, while the observed number of organs transplanted refers to the number of organs that were actually transplanted.

ORPD: Organs recovered per donor, a statistic computed by dividing the total number of organs recovered by the total number of donors. For this calculation, the number of donors is not limited to donors who had eligible deaths.

OTPD: Organs transplanted per donor, a statistic computed by dividing the total number of organs transplanted by the number of donors. For this calculation, the number of donors is not limited to those with eligible deaths.

Oviedo Convention: Officially the *Convention for the Protection of Human Rights and Dignity of the Human Being with regard to the Application of*

Biology and Medicine, a framework that entered into force in 1999 and that which includes a protocol addressing issues in human organ donation and transplantation.

Pancreas: A gland that performs various functions, including secretion of insulin and digestive enzymes.

Peritoneal dialysis: A process of filtering body wastes by filling the abdomen with a solution called dialysate that helps to remove toxins. These fluids are retained in the abdomen for some time and then drained out, allowing the inside lining of the individual's belly acting as a natural filter.

Potential Donor Audit: In the United Kingdom, an audit completed by specialist nurses to determine the number of potential donors of solid organs in the United Kingdom and to collect information as to why some patients did not become organ donors.

Presumed consent: A system in which it is assumed that a deceased person has granted permission for their organs and tissues to be donated, unless they have indicated otherwise. Presumed consent is also known as an "opt-out" system, because people must explicitly state that they wish to not participate in organ donation.

Procurement: The process of removing tissues, organs, or other body parts from a donor.

Procurement coordinator: An individual responsible for discussing organ donation with family members, evaluating potential donors, managing the donor during the recovery of organs, and arranging for the organ donation process. A procurement coordinator is usually a medically trained person, often a nurse.

Qualifying relationship: A relationship that designates a person who can indicate whether a deceased person's organs can be donated, in the absence of any indication from the deceased person themselves regarding their wishes. Normally, consent for donation must be obtained from the highest ranked person on the list of qualifying relationships. In the United States, the *Human Tissues Act of 2004* indicates the following ranked list of qualifying relationships: spouse or partner, parent or child, brother or sister, grandparent or grandchild, niece or nephew, stepfather or stepmother, half-sibling, friend of long standing.

Recovery: The process of removing organs or tissues from a donor's body.

Required referral: A system in which all deaths and anticipated deaths are referred to a health care professional who is responsible for organ donation. All hospitals in the United States must have a required referral system and must notify the local organ procurement organization of deaths.

Required request: A stipulation that hospitals have a system to ask the families of all potential donors to donate the organs and tissues of a deceased family member. The United States passed a law stipulating the required request in 1986, with the purpose of increasing the number of donations.

Scientific Registry of Transplant Recipients (SRTR): A registry created in the United States in 1984 as part of the National Organ Transplant Act. The purpose of the Scientific Registry of Transplant Recipients is to provide information about organ transplants, including patient and graft survival rates and clinical information about donors, transplant candidates, and transplant recipients.

Solid organ transplants: Transplants of organs such as the heart, intestines, kidney, liver, lung, and pancreas.

Status: The degree of medical urgency for patients on a waiting list for organ transplants.

Stem cell transplants: Transplants in which stem cells are infused into a patient's blood stream. Stem cell transplants are used to treat numerous conditions, including lymphoma, immunodeficiency, and the side effects of chemotherapy.

Time on waiting list: The length of time that passes between an individual being placed on a wait list for an organ transplant and their receipt of an organ or removal from the wait list for other reasons.

Tissue: Part of the human body made up of cells with a similar structure and which perform a specific type of function; besides the cells, body tissues include the intercellular matrix, which fills the spaces between cells. Examples of tissues in the human body include corneas, veins, bones, muscles, and tendons. As cells combine to make body tissues, so tissues combine to make body organs.

Tissue typing: Also called histocompatibility, the process of testing for antigens to see if a donor organ will be accepted by the potential recipient's body.

Transplant candidate: An individual who has been placed on the waiting list for an organ donation and is eligible to receive a transplanted organ or organs should a suitable organ or organs become available.

Transplant commercialism: The treatment of organs, tissues, or cells as a commodity that can be bought and sold or otherwise used for material gain.

Transplant tourism: Travel for the purpose of obtaining an organ transplant, sometimes in connection with organ trafficking or transplant commercialism.

United Network for Organ Sharing: The organization in the United States that operates the Organ Procurement and Transplantation Network (OPTN).

Utilized donor: A person from whom one or more organs has been recovered for transplant and one or more of those organs is actually used for transplant.

Vascularized Composite Allograft (VCA): A transplant that includes multiple types of tissues; examples of VCAs include face and hand transplants.

Vitrification: A cryopreservation technique that uses cryoprotectant concentrations to prevent crystallization while producing a glass-like solidification of the material being preserved.

Waiting list: A list of individuals who have registered and are waiting for a donated organ or other cells or tissues.

Xenograft: An organ or tissue procured from a member of one species and transplanted into a member of another, for instance, an organ from a pig transplanted into a person.

DIRECTORY OF RESOURCES

BOOKS

Beard, T. Randolph, David L. Kaserman, and Rigmar Ostercamp. *The global organ shortage: Economic causes, human consequences, policy responses.* Stanford, CA: Stanford Economics and Finance/Stanford University Press, 2013.

Ben-David, Oril Brawer. *Organ donation and transplantation: Body organs as an exchangeable socio-cultural resource.* Westport, CT: Praeger, 2005.

Boas, Hagai, Yael Hashiloni-Dolev, Nadav Davidovitch, Dani Filc, and Shai Lavi, eds. *Bioethics and biopolitics in Israel: Socio-legal, political and empirical analysis.* New York: Cambridge University Press, 2018.

Brezina, Corona. *Organ donation: Risks, rewards, and research.* New York: The Rosen Publishing Group, 2010.

Childress, James F., Sarah Domnitz, and Catharyn T. Liverman, eds. *Opportunities for organ donation research: Saving lives by improving the quality and quantity of organs for transplantation.* Washington, DC: The National Academics Press, 2017.

Cohen, I. Glenn. *Patients with passports: Medical tourism, law and ethics.* New York: Oxford University Press, 2015.

Crowley-Matoka, Megan. *Domesticating organ transplant: Familial sacrifice and national aspiration in Mexico.* Durham, NC: Duke University Press, 2016.

DeMicco, Frederick J., ed. *Medical tourism and wellness: Hospitality bridging healthcare.* Toronto: Apple Academic Press, 2017.

Farrell, Anne-Maree, David Price, and Muireann Quigley. *Organ shortage: Ethics, law, and pragmatism.* New York: Cambridge University Press, 2011.

Fry-Revere, Sigrid. *The kidney sellers: A journey of discovery in Iran.* Durham, NC: Carolina Academic Press, 2014.

Gray, Sarah. *A life everlasting: The extraordinary story of one boy's gift to medical science*. New York: HarperOne, 2016.

Hamilton, David. *A history of organ transplantation: Ancient legends to modern practice*. Pittsburgh, PA: University of Pittsburgh Press, 2012.

Herring, Jonathan. *Medical law and ethics*. 4th ed. Oxford: Oxford University Press, 2012.

Holland, Stephen. *Bioethics: A philosophical introduction*. Malden, MA: Polity, 2017.

Ishiguro, Kazuo. *Never let me go*. London: Faber and Faber, 2005.

Issenberg, Sasha. *Outpatients: The astonishing new world of medical tourism*. New York: Columbia Global Reports, 2016.

Jox, Ralf J., Galia Asssadi, and Georg Marckmann, eds. *Organ transplantation in times of donor shortage: Challenges and solutions*. Cham, Switzerland: Springer, 2016.

Kochen, Madeline. *Organ donation and the divine lien in Talmudic law*. New York: Cambridge University Press, 2014.

Meilaender, Gilbert. *Bioethics: A primer for Christians*. 3rd ed. Grand Rapids, MI: William B. Eerdmans Pub. Co., 2013.

Mezrich, Joshua D. *When death becomes life: Notes from a transplant surgeon*. New York: HarperCollins, 2019.

Miller, Franklin G., and Robert D. Truog. *Death, dying, and organ transplantation: Reconstructing medical ethics at the end of life*. Oxford: Oxford University Press, 2012.

Mosher, Lucinda. *Personhood, illness and death in America's multifaith neighborhoods: A practical guide*. London: Jessica Kingsley Publishers, 2018.

Russell, Emily. *Transplant fictions: A cultural study of organ exchange*. Cham, Switzerland: Palgrave Macmillan, 2019.

Saidi, Reza F., ed. *Organ donation and organ donors: Issues, challenges, and perspectives*. New York: Nova Biomedical, 2013.

Shaw, Bud. *Last night in the OR: A transplant surgeon's odyssey*. New York: Plume, 2015.

Siegel, Jason T., and Eusebio M. Alvaro. *Understanding organ donation: Applied behavioral science perspectives*. Malden, MA: Wiley-Blackwell, 2010.

U.S. Department of Health & Human Services. Scientific Registry of Transplant Recipients. *2018 OPTN/SRTR Annual Data Report*. Rockville, MD: Department of Health and Human Services, Health Resources and Services Administration, 2018. https://srtr.transplant.hrsa.gov/annual_reports/2018_ADR_Preview.aspx (accessed 26 Oct. 2020).

Van Brussel, Leen, and Nico Carpentier, eds. *The social construction of death: Interdisciplinary perspectives*. New York: Palgrave Macmillan, 2014.

ARTICLES

Abouna, George M. (2003). "Ethical Issues in Organ Transplantation." *Medical Principles and Practice 12*: 54–69. https://www.karger.com/Article/Pdf/68158 (accessed 21 Dec. 2019).

Adams, M. P. (2017). "The ethics of organ tourism: Role morality and organ transplantation." *The Journal of Medicine and Philosophy* 42(6): 670–689.

Aleccia, JoNel, and Kaiser Health News (2018). "'Wallet biopsy': Organ transplant often depends on patient's finances." *CNN.com* (24 Dec. 2018). https://www.cnn.com/2018/12/24/health/organ-transplant-center-payment-partner/index.html (accessed 23 Jan. 2021).

Arshad, Adam, Benjamin Anderson, and Adnan Sharif (2019). "Comparison of organ donation and transplantation between opt-out and opt-in systems." *Kidney International* 95: 1453–1460. https://www.kidney-international.org/article/S0085-2538(19)30185-1/fulltext (accessed 27 Oct. 2020).

Ashkenazi, Tamar, Jacob Lavee, and Eytan Mor. (2015). "Organ donation in Israel—Achievements and challenges." *Transplantation* 99(2): 265–266.

Australian Government. Department of Health (n.d.). "Supporting living organ donors program" [website]. https://www.health.gov.au/initiatives-and-programs/supporting-living-organ-donors-program (accessed 5 Nov. 2020).

Bai, Ge, and Gerard F. Anderson (2016). "US hospitals are still using charge-master markups to maximize revenues." *Health Affairs* 35(9): 1658–1664. https://www.healthaffairs.org/doi/pdf/10.1377/hlthaff.2016.0093 (accessed 2 Nov. 2020).

Barker, C. F., and J. F. Markmann (2013). "Historical overview of transplantation." *Cold Spring Harbor perspectives in medicine 3*(4): a014977. http://perspectives inmedicine.cshlp.org/content/3/4/a014977.full (accessed 11 Nov. 2019).

Bengali, Shashank, and Ramin Mostaghim (2017). "'Kidney for sale': Iran has a legal market for the organs, but the system doesn't always work." *Los Angeles Times* (15 Oct. 2017). https://www.latimes.com/world/middleeast/la-fg-iran-kidney-20171015-story.html (accessed 19 Dec. 2019).

Bentley, T. Scott, and Nick J. Ortner (2020). "2020 U.S. organ and tissue transplants: Cost estimates, discussion, and emerging issues." *Milliman Research Report* (Jan. 2020). https://www.milliman.com/-/media/milliman/pdfs/articles/2020-us-organ-tissue-transplants.ashx (accessed 2 Nov. 2020).

Bezinover, D., and F. Saner (2019). "Organ transplantation in the modern era." *BMC anesthesiology 19*(1): 32. https://www.ncbi.nlm.nih.gov/pmc/articles/PMC6399965/ (accessed 11 Nov. 2019).

Bigg, Clair (2016) "'Gutted like a pig': Grieving mother takes on Russia's organ donation system." *Radio Free Europe/ Radio Liberty* (16 Mar. 2016). https://www.rferl.org/a/russia-organ-harvesting-grieving-mother/27617168.html (accessed 26 Apr. 2020).

Boodman, Eric (2018). "A 'breakthrough in organ preservation': Study shows keeping livers warm helps preserve them for transplant." *Statnews* (18 Apr. 2018). https://www.statnews.com/2018/04/18/lung-transplant-technology/ (accessed 1 Apr. 2020).

Brasor, Philip (2017). "Organ donations and transplants still face obstacles in Japan." *The Japan Times* (28 Oct. 2017). https://www.japantimes.co.jp

/news/2017/10/28/national/media-national/organ-donations-transplants
-still-face-obstacles-japan/#.Xf5Kny2ZMU0 (accessed 21 Dec. 2019).

Brody, Jane E. (1995). "Questions are raised on Mantle Transplant." *The New York Times* (2 Aug. 1995).

Bruzzone, Pierluigi (2008). "Religious aspects of organ transplantation." *Transplantation Proceedings* 40(4): 1064–1067.

Caplan, Arthur, and Brendan Parent (n.d.). "Organ transplantation." The Hastings Center: Bioethics Briefings. https://www.thehastingscenter.org/publications -resources/hastings-center-bioethics-briefings/ (accessed 12 Nov. 2020).

China Organ Harvest Research Center (2019). "Documenting genocide: The extrajudicial killing of prisoners of conscience for organs in China and the campaign to eradicate Falun Gong: Factual findings & analysis report." https://www.chinaorganharvest.org/app/uploads/2019/04/COHRC-Factual -Findings-Report.pdf (accessed 1 Nov. 2020).

China Organ Harvest Research Center (n.d.). "Legislation" [web page]. https:// www.chinaorganharvest.org/legislation/ (accessed 1 Nov. 2020).

China Organ Harvest Research Center (n.d.). "Resolutions" [web page]. https:// www.chinaorganharvest.org/resolutions/ (accessed 1 Nov. 2020).

The China Tribunal (2020). "China tribunal full judgment." (March 2020). https://chinatribunal.com/wp-content/uploads/2020/03/ChinaTribunal _JUDGMENT_1stMarch_2020.pdf (accessed 31 Oct. 2020).

Cooper, David K. C., Burcin Ekser, and A. Joseph Tector (2015). "A brief history of clinical xenotransplantation." *International Journal of Surgery* 23 (Part B): 205–210. https://www.ncbi.nlm.nih.gov/pmc/articles/PMC4684730/ (accessed 2 May 2020).

Crawford, Todd C., Trent Magruder, Joshua C. Grimm, Alejandro Suarez-Pierre, Nishant Patel, Christopher M. Sciortino, John V. Conte, Robert S. Higgins, Duke E. Camerson, and Glenn J. Whitman (2018). "A comprehensive risk score to predict prolonged hospital stay after heart transplantation." *The Annals of Thoracic Surgery* 105: 83–91. https://www.annalsthoracicsurgery .org/article/S0003-4975(17)31037-8/pdf (accessed 5 Apr. 2020).

David, Ashley E., Sanjay Mehrotra, Lisa M. McElroy, John J. Friedewald, Anton I. Scaro, Brittany Lapin, Raymond Kang, Jane L. Holl, Michael M. Abecassis, and Daniela P. Ladner (2014). "The extend and predictors of waiting time geographic disparity in kidney transplantation in the United States." *Transplantation* 97(10):1049–1057.

Davidai, Shai, Thomas Gilovich, and Lee D. Ross (2012). "The meaning of default options for potential organ donors." *Proceedings of the National Academy of Sciences* 109(38): 15201–15205. https://www.pnas.org/content /109/38/15201 (accessed 27 Oct. 2020).

Denyer, Simon (2017). "China used to harvest organs from prisoners. Under pressure, that practice is finally ending." *The Washington Post* (15 Sept. 2017). https://www.washingtonpost.com/world/asia_pacific/in-the-face-of-criticism

-china-has-been-cleaning-up-its-organ-transplant-industry/2017/09/14
/d689444e-e1a2-11e6-a419-eefe8eff0835_story.html (accessed 31 Oct. 2020).

Dominguez-Gil, Beatriz, ed. "Newsletter transplant: International figures on donation and transplantation 2018." Global Observatory on Donation and Transplantation (updated 12 Sept. 2019). http://www.transplant-observatory.org/download/newsletter-transplant-2019/ (accessed 11 Nov. 2019).

Enderby, Cher, and Ceasar A. Keller (2015). "An overview of immunosuppression in solid organ transplantation." *American Journal of Managed Care* 21: S12–S23. https://www.ajmc.com/journals/supplement/2015/ace022_jan15
_organtransplant_ce/ace022_jan15_enderby (accessed 6 Apr. 2020).

European Parliament. Directorate-General for External Policies. Policy Department. (2015). "Trafficking in human origins." https://www.europarl.europa.eu/RegData/etudes/STUD/2015/549055/EXPO_STU(2015)549055
_EN.pdf (accessed 30 Oct. 2020).

Feeley, Thomas Hugh, and Shin-Il Moon (2009). "Promoting organ donations through public education campaigns: A random-effects meta-analysis." *Communication Reports* 22(2): 63–73. https://www.organdonor.gov/sites/default
/files/about-dot/files/metaanalysisfinalmanuscript.pdf (accessed 28 Oct. 2020).

Ghods, Ahad J., and Shekoufeh Savaj (2006). "Iranian model of paid and regulated living-unrelated kidney donation." *ASN Kidney News* 1(6): 1136–1145. https://cjasn.asnjournals.org/content/1/6/1136 (accessed 5 Nov. 2020).

Giwa, Sebastian, Jebediah K. Lewis, Luis Alvarez, Robert Langer, Alvin E. Roth, et al. (2017). "The promise of organ and tissue preservation to transform medicine." *Nature Biotechnology* 35:530–542. https://www.nature.com/articles
/nbt.3889 (accessed 26 Oct. 2020).

Glazier, Alexandra K. (Aug. 2018). "Organ donation and the principles of gift law." *CJASN: Clinical Journal of the American Society of Nephrology* 13(3): 1283–1284. https://cjasn.asnjournals.org/content/13/8/1283 (accessed 18 Dec 2019).

Hawkins, K. C., A. Scales, P. Murphy, S. Madden, and J. Brierly (2017). "Current status of paediatric and neonatal organ donation in the UK." *Archives of Disease in Childhood 103*: 210–215.

Health Resources and Services Administration Newsroom (2020). "New rule expands the scope of reimbursable expenses for living organ donation." https://www.hrsa.gov/about/news/press-releases/new-rule-expands-scope
-living-organ-donation (accessed 5 Nov. 2020).

Hennessey, Jaime J. (2006). "A members-only club for organ donors." Abcnews.go.com (9 Dec. 2006). https://abcnews.go.com/Health/story?id=2071084
&page=1 (accessed 28 Oct. 2020).

Hippen, Benjamin, Lainie Friedman Ross, and Robert M. Sade (2010). "Saving lives is more important than abstract moral concerns: Incentives should be used to increase organ donation." *Annals of Thoracic Surgery* 88(4): 1053–1061.

https://www.ncbi.nlm.nih.gov/pmc/articles/PMC2766511/ (accessed 5 Nov. 2020).

"Implantable artificial kidney achieves pre-clinical milestone." *Science Daily* (7 Nov. 2019). https://www.sciencedaily.com/releases/2019/11/191107170503 .htm (accessed 2 May 2020).

Israni, A. K., D. Zaun, J. D. Rosendale, C. Schaffhausen, J. J. Snyder, and B. L. Kasiske. (27 Feb. 2019). "OPTN/SRTR 2017 annual data report: Deceased organ donation." *American Journal of Transplantation* 19(2): 485–517. https://onlinelibrary.wiley.com/doi/full/10.1111/ajt.15280 (accessed 19 Dec. 2019).

Jing, Lei, Leeann Yao, Michael Zhao, Li-ping Peng, and Mingyao Liu (2018). "Organ preservation: From the past to the future." *Acta Pharmacologica Sinica* 39(5): 845–857. https://www.ncbi.nlm.nih.gov/pmc/articles /PMC5943901/ (accessed 1 Apr. 2020).

"John Hunter: 'Founder of Scientific Surgery.'" *Hematology/Oncology Today* (25 Jan. 2009). https://www.healio.com/hematology-oncology/news/print /hemonc-today/%7Bc9a8ca57-fa27-4432-aadf-d8ee0671428f%7D/john -hunter-founder-of-scientific-surgery (accessed 11 Nov. 2019).

Johns Hopkins Medicine News Release (2012). "Younger patients more likely to live a decade or longer after heart transplant." (Feb. 27, 2012). https://www .hopkinsmedicine.org/news/media/releases/younger_patients_more_likely _to_live_a_decade_or_longer_after_heart_transplant (accessed 12 Apr. 2020).

Kahn, Chip (2015). "Words matter: Defining hospital charges, costs, and payments—and the number that matter most." *Federal of American Hospitals Policy Blog* (5 June 2015). https://www.fah.org/blog/words-matter-defining -hospital-charges-costs-and-payments-and-the-numbers-t (accessed 2 Nov. 2020).

Krishna, Murali, and Peter Lepping (2011). "Ethical debate: Ethics of xeno-transplantation." *British Journal of Medical Practitioners* 4(3): a425. https:// www.bjmp.org/files/2011-4-3/bjmp-2011-4-3-a425.pdf (accessed 10 Nov. 2020).

Labrecque, Michelle, R. Parad, M. Gupta, and A. Hansen (2011). "Donation after cardiac death: The potential contribution of an infant donor population." *The Journal of Pediatrics 158*(1): 31–36.

"The littlest donors: Neonatal donation offers hope in tragedy." *NBC News* (18 Mar. 2014). https://www.nbcnews.com/health/kids-health/littlest-donors -neonatal-organ-donation-offers-hope-tragedy-n51436 (accessed 21 Dec. 2019).

Low, Harry (2017). "My son died in 1994 but his heart only stopped beating this year." *BBC News* (4 May 2017). https://www.bbc.com/news /magazine-39422660. (accessed 28 Oct. 2020).

MacDonald, Anna (2019). "Bioprinting organs: A future Alternative to Organ Donation?" *Technology Networks* (2 Sept. 2019). https://www.technology networks.com/cell-science/articles/bioprinting-organs-a-future-alternative -to-organ-donation-323422 (accessed 2 May 2020).

Major, Rupert W. L. (2008). "Paying kidney donors: time to follow Iran?" *McGill Journal of Medicine* 11(1): 67–69. https://www.ncbi.nlm.nih.gov/pmc/articles/PMC2322914/

Martin, Dominique E., Kristof Van Assche, Beatriz Dominguez-Gil, Marta Lopez-Fraga, Rudolf Garcia Gallont, Elmi Muller, Eric Rondeau, and Alexander M. Capron (2019). "A new edition of the Declaration of Istanbul: updated guidance to combat organ trafficking and transplant tourism worldwide." *Kidney International* 95:757–759. https://www.kidney-international.org/article/S0085-2538(19)30033-X/pdf (accessed 30 Oct. 2020).

Matas, David, and David Kilgour (2006). "Report into allegations of organ harvesting of Falun Gong practitioners in China." (6 July 2006). http://www.david-kilgour.com/2006/Kilgour-Matas-organ-harvesting-rpt-July6-eng.pdf (accessed 31 Oct. 2020).

Min, Lim (2018). "Living organ donation in Singapore." *Asia Law Network* (5 Dec. 2018). https://learn.asialawnetwork.com/2018/12/05/living-organ-donation-in-singapore/ (accessed 5 Nov. 2020).

Movesian, Matthew (2016). "Should doctors game the transplant wait list to help their patients?" Shots: Health News from NPR (24 July 2016). https://www.npr.org/sections/health-shots/2016/07/24/486787474/should-doctors-game-the-transplant-wait-list-to-help-their-patients (accessed 12 Nov. 2020).

New Zealand Government. Science Learning Hub. "History of xenotransplantation." https://www.sciencelearn.org.nz/resources/1214-history-of-xenotransplantation (accessed 2 May 2020).

Norris, Sonya. (2018a). "Consent for organ donation in Canada." *HillNotes: Research and Analysis from Canada's Library of Parliament* (23 Jan. 2018). https://hillnotes.ca/2018/01/23/consent-for-organ-donation-in-canada/ (accessed 19 Dec. 2019).

Norris, Sonya (2018b). "Organ donation and transplantation in Canada: Background paper." Library of Parliament Research Papers Publication No. 2018-13-E. Ottawa, Canada: Library of Parliament, 2018. https://lop.parl.ca/staticfiles/PublicWebsite/Home/ResearchPublications/BackgroundPapers/PDF/2018-13-e.pdf (accessed 19 Dec. 2019).

"Organ bioprinting gets a breath of fresh air." *ScienceDaily* (May 2, 2019). https://www.sciencedaily.com/releases/2019/05/190502143518.htm (accessed 2 May 2020).

Organ Procurement and Transplantation Network (4 Feb. 2020). "New national liver and intestinal organ transplant system in effect." https://unos.org/news/new-national-liver-and-intestinal-organ-transplant-system-in-effect-feb-4-2020/ (accessed 4 Apr. 2020).

Ossola, Alexandra (2017). "Crisis in America: Medical experts use new tech tools to combat the organ transplant shortage." *CNBC: Modern Medicine* (21 June 2017). https://www.cnbc.com/2017/06/20/medical-experts-use-new-tech-tools-to-combat-organ-transplant-shortage.html (accessed 21 Dec. 2019).

Pischke, Sven, Marie C. Lege, Moritz von Wulffen, Antonio Galante, Benjamin Otto, Malte H. Wehmeyer, Uta Herden, Lutz Fischer, Björm Nashan, Ansgar W. Lohse, and Martina Sterneck. (2017). "Factors associated with long-term survival after liver transplantation: A retrospective cohort study." *World Journal of Hepatology* 9(8): 427–435. https://www.ncbi.nlm.nih.gov/pmc/articles/PMC5355765/ (accessed 12 Apr. 2020).

Pope Francis (Jorge Mario Bergoglio) (13 Apr. 2019). "Address of his holiness Pope Francis to the Italian Association for the Donation of Organs, Tissues and Cells (AIDO)." *Libreria Editrice Vaticana*. http://www.vatican.va/content/francesco/en/speeches/2019/april/documents/papa-francesco_20190413_donazione-organi.html (accessed 22 Apr. 2020).

Pullen, Lara C. (28 May 2019). "Tackling the growing problem of transporting organs." *American Journal of Transplantation* 19: 1603–1604. https://onlinelibrary.wiley.com/doi/full/10.1111/ajt.15410 (accessed 4 Apr. 2020).

Ross, Lainie Friedman, Richard Thistlewaite, and the Committee of Bioethics (2008). "Minors as solid living-organ donors." American Academy of Pediatrics: Clinical Reports 2008-1525. https://pediatrics.aappublications.org/content/pediatrics/122/2/454.full.pdf (accessed 21 Dec. 2019).

Schaubel, D. E., M. K. Guidinger, S. W. Biggins, J. D. Kalbfleisch, E. A. Pomfret, P. Sharma, and R. M. Merion (2009). "Survival benefit-based deceased-donor liver allocation." *American Journal of Transplantation* 9(4 Pt 2): 970–981.

Sickand, Manisha, M. S. Cuerden, S. W. Klarenbach, A. O. Ojo, C. R. Parikh, N. Boudville, and A. X. Garg (2009). "Reimbursing live organ donors for incurred non-medical expenses: A global perspective on policies and programs." *American Journal of Transplantation* 9(12): 2825–2836. https://onlinelibrary.wiley.com/doi/full/10.1111/j.1600-6143.2009.02829.x (accessed 5 Nov. 2020).

Simpson, P. J. (Jan. 2012). "What are the issues in organ donation in 2012?" *British Journal of Anaesthesia*, 108(Suppl_1): i3–i6. https://academic.oup.com/bja/article/108/suppl_1/i3/237272 (accessed 21 Dec. 2019).

Southard, James H., and Folkert O. Belzer (Feb 1995). "Organ preservation." *Annual Review of Medicine* 46. https://www.annualreviews.org/doi/pdf/10.1146/annurev.med.46.1.235 (accessed 1 Apr. 2020).

Starzl Institute, UPMC (2020) "Weaning transplant recipients from immunosuppressive drugs." https://www.upmc.com/services/transplant/about/starzl-institute/drug-weaning (accessed 6 Apr. 2020).

Thabut, Gabriel, and Herve Mal (2017). "Outcomes after lung transplantation." *Journal of Thoracic Disease* 9(8):2684–2691. http://jtd.amegroups.com/article/view/14758/html (accessed 12 Apr. 2020).

Tibell, Annika (2007). "The transplantation society's policy on interaction with China." *Doctors Against Forced Organ Harvesting* [website] (Aug. 15, 2007). https://dafoh.org/the-transplantation-societys-policy-on-interactions-with-china/ (accessed 31 Oct. 2020).

"Transplant Tourism: A 'pervasive' and dangerous 'shadow world of medicine.'" *Infectious Disease News* (Apr. 2019). https://www.healio.com/news/infectious-disease/20190416/transplant-tourism-a-pervasive-and-dangerous-shadow-world-of-medicine (accessed 30 Oct. 2020).

Tsai, Daniel Fu-Chang, Shei-Wei Huang, Soren Holm, Pi-Yi Lin, Yu-Kang Chang, and Chih-Cheng Hsu. (2017). "The outcomes and controversies of transplant tourism—Lessons of an 11-year retrospective cohort study from Taiwan." *PLoS ONE* 12(6): e0178569. https://journals.plos.org/plosone/article?id=10.1371/journal.pone.0178569 (accessed 30 Oct. 2020).

United Nations Office on Drugs and Crime (2014). "Global report on trafficking in persons." https://www.unodc.org/documents/data-and-analysis/glotip/GLOTIP_2014_full_report.pdf (accessed 30 Oct. 2020).

United Network for Organ Sharing (2020). "Contacting my donor family." https://transplantliving.org/community/contacting-my-donor-family/ (accessed 12 Nov. 2020).

United Network for Organ Sharing (2020). "Transplant trends." https://unos.org/data/transplant-trends/ (accessed 26 Oct. 2020).

United Network for Organ Sharing (n.d.). "Covering costs." https://transplantliving.org/financing-a-transplant/ (accessed 3 Nov. 2020).

University of California-Davis Health: Transplant Center (2020). "Donation after cardiac death (DCD)." https://health.ucdavis.edu/transplant/nonlivingdonors/donation-after-cardiac-death.html (accessed 9 Nov. 2020).

U.S. Food & Drug Administration (2019). "Xenotransplantation." https://www.fda.gov/vaccines-blood-biologics/xenotransplantation (accessed 10 Nov. 2020).

Weiss, Matthew J., Alicia Pérez Blanco, and Ben Gelbart (Mar. 2019). "Special issues in pediatric deceased organ donation." *Intensive Care Medicine* 45(3): 363. https://link.springer.com/article/10.1007/s00134-019-05523-2 (accessed 21 Dec. 2019).

World Health Organization (2005). "Statement from the Xenotransplantation Advisory Consultation." (18–20 Apr. 2005). https://www.who.int/transplantation/XenoEnglish.pdf?ua=1 (accessed 2 May 2020).

Zaltzman, Jeffrey (Aug. 2018). "Ten years of Israel's organ transplant law: Is it on the right track?" *Israel Journal of Health Policy Research* 7(45). https://ijhpr.biomedcentral.com/articles/10.1186/s13584-018-0232-1 (accessed 19 Dec. 2019).

ORGANIZATIONS

American Association of Tissue Banks https://www.aatb.org/
American Foundation for Donation and Transplantation https://www.afdt.org/
American Society of Transplant Surgeons https://asts.org/
American Society of Transplantation https://www.myast.org/
Association for Multicultural Affairs in Transplantation http://www.amat1.org/

Association of Organ Procurement Organizations https://www.aopo.org/

Australia and New Zealand Organ Donation Registry (ANZOD) https://www.anzdata.org.au/anzod/

Blood & Marrow Transplant Information Network https://www.bmtinfonet.org/

Canadian Blood Services https://blood.ca/en/organs-tissues

Canadian Donation and Transplantation Research Program https://www.cntrp.ca/

Canadian Transplant Society https://www.cantransplant.ca/organ/

Chris Klug Foundation https://chrisklugfoundation.org/

Donate Life America https://www.donatelife.net/

Donation for Research (Center for Organ Recovery and Education) https://www.core.org/understanding-donation/donation-for-research/

EFRETOS: European Framework for the Evaluation of Organ Transplantation https://eurotransplant.org/cms/index.php?page=efretos

Eurotransplant https://www.eurotransplant.org/cms/

Eye Bank Association of America https://restoresight.org/

FOEDUS: Fostering Exchange of Organs Donated in EU Member States https://www.foedus-eoeo.eu/#/public

International Registry in Organ Donation and Transplantation http://www.irodat.org/

International Society for Heart and Lung Transplantation https://ishlt.org/

National Donor Family Council https://www.kidney.org/transplantation/donorfamilies

National Marrow Donor Program https://bethematch.org/

National Minority Organ Tissue Transplant Education Program https://www.natlmottep.org/

North American Transplant Coordinator's Organization http://www.natco1.org/home/index.asp

ODEQUS: Organ Donation European Quality System http://www.odequs.eu

Organ Donation and Transplantation Alliance https://organdonationalliance.org/

Organ Procurement and Transplantation Network https://optn.transplant.hrsa.gov/

Scientific Registry of Transplant Recipients https://www.srtr.org/

Southwest Transplant Alliance https://organ.org/

Transplant Quebec https://www.transplantquebec.ca/en/organ-donation-and-transplantation-quebec

TRIO: Transplant Recipients International Organization https://www.trioweb.org/

UNOS: United Network for Organ Sharing https://unos.org/

WEBSITES

Allocation Calculators (U.S. Department of Health & Human Services) https://optn.transplant.hrsa.gov/resources/allocation-calculators/

Canadian Blood Services: Organs & Tissues for Life https://blood.ca/en/organs-tissues

Canadian Institute for Health Information: Organ replacement in Canada: CORR annual statistics, 2019 https://www.cihi.ca/en/organ-replacement-in-canada-corr-annual-statistics-2019

Council of Europe: Organ Donation and Transplantation https://www.coe.int/en/web/human-rights-channel/organ-donation

Declaration of Istanbul on Organ Trafficking and Transplant Tourism https://www.declarationofistanbul.org/

Directive 2010/45/EU of the European Parliament and of the Council of 7 July 2010 (the European Organs Directive) https://eur-lex.europa.eu/legal-content/EN/TXT/?uri=CELEX:02010L0053-20100806

Donate Life: Australian Government Organ and Tissue Authority https://donatelife.gov.au/

Ethical Principles in the Allocation of Human Organs (U.S. Department of Health & Human Services) https://optn.transplant.hrsa.gov/resources/ethics/ethical-principles-in-the-allocation-of-human-organs/

European Commission: Blood, Tissues, Cells and Organs https://ec.europa.eu/health/blood_tissues_organs/organs_en

Federal and States Laws About Living Donation (American Society of Transplantation) http://www.livedonortoolkit.com/financial-toolkit/federal-and-state-laws-about-living-donation

Human Organ Transplantation (World Health Organization) https://www.who.int/transplantation/organ/en/

Living Donation (United Network for Organ Sharing) https://unos.org/transplant/living-donation/

Living Donor Liver Transplantation FAQs (Columbia University Center for Liver Disease and Transplantation) https://columbiasurgery.org/liver/living-donor-liver-transplantation-faqs

Living-donor Transplant (Mayo Clinic) https://www.mayoclinic.org/tests-procedures/living-donor-transplant/about/pac-20384787

Medline Plus: Organ donation (National Library of Medicine) https://medlineplus.gov/organdonation.html

National Health Service (England): Organ donation and your beliefs: Religious perspectives on organ donation https://www.organdonation.nhs.uk/helping-you-to-decide/your-faith-and-beliefs/

National Health Service: Organ Donation (England) https://www.organdonation.nhs.uk/

Organ Donation and Transplantation (Health Resources and Services Administration, U.S.) https://data.hrsa.gov/topics/health-systems/organ-donation

Organ donation and transplantation: Policy Actions at the EU Level https://ec.europa.eu/health/blood_tissues_organs/consultations/policy_options/oc_organs_en

Organ Donation FAQs (Health Resources & Services Administration) https://www.organdonor.gov/about/facts-terms/donation-faqs.html

Organ Procurement and Transplantation Network: National Data https://optn.transplant.hrsa.gov/data/view-data-reports/national-data/

Organ Transport (U.S. Department of Health & Human Services) https://optn.transplant.hrsa.gov/resources/organ-transport/

Pediatric Transplant (U.S. Department of Health & Human Services) https://optn
.transplant.hrsa.gov/resources/pediatric-transplant/

Statistics and Stories: Organ Donation (Health Resources and Services Administration, U.S.) https://www.organdonor.gov/statistics-stories.html

Theological perspectives on organ donation (United Network for Organ Sharing) https://unos.org/transplant/facts/theological-perspective-on-organ-and
-tissue-donation/

Transplant Safety (Centers for Disease Control and Prevention) https://www.cdc
.gov/transplantsafety/overview/key-facts.html

Transweb: A Resource on Transplantation and Donation (University of Michigan
Transplant Center http://www.transweb.org/index.shtml

World Health Organization Guiding Principles on Human Cell, Tissue, and Organ
Transplantation https://www.who.int/transplantation/Guiding_Principles
Transplantation_WHA63.22en.pdf?ua=1

Xenotransplantation (U.S. Food and Drug Administration) https://www.fda.gov
/vaccines-blood-biologics/xenotransplantation

Xenotransplantation (World Health Organization) https://www.who.int/transplan
tation/xeno/en/

INDEX

About the Author

Sarah Boslaugh, PhD, MPH, is a professional tutor in mathematics and economics at Forest Park Community College in Saint Louis, Missouri. She received her PhD in Measurement and Evaluation from the Graduate Center of the City University of New York and her MPH from Saint Louis University. Her other books include *Secondary Data Sources for Public Health: A Practical Guide* (2007); *Statistics in a Nutshell* (2nd ed, 2012); *Health Care Systems Around the World: A Comparative Guide* (2013); and, for ABC-CLIO, *Drug Resistance* (2016), *Transgender Health Issues* (2018), and *Genetic Testing* (2020). She also served as editor-in-chief for *Encyclopedia of Epidemiology* (2008) and *The SAGE Encyclopedia of Pharmacology and Society* (2015).